Nuclear Medicine Physics

The Basics

Fifth Edition

Nuclear Medicine Physics

The Basics

Fifth Edition

Ramesh Chandra, PhD
Professor
Department of Radiology
New York University Medical Center
New York, New York

Williams & Wilkins
A WAVERLY COMPANY

BALTIMORE • PHILADELPHIA • LONDON • PARIS • BANGKOK
BUENOS AIRES • HONG KONG • MUNICH • SYDNEY • TOKYO • WROCLAW

Editor: Charles W. Mitchell
Managing Editor: Grace E. Miller
Marketing Manager: Lorraine A. Smith
Production Coordinator: Felecia R. Weber
Project Editor: Bill Cady
Freelance Copy Editor: Pam Thomson
Illustration Planner: Lorraine Wrzosek
Typesetter: Peirce Graphic Services, Inc.
Printer and Binder: Port City Press, Inc.

351 West Camden Street
Baltimore, Maryland 21201-2436 USA

Rose Tree Corporate Center
1400 North Providence Road
Building II, Suite 5025
Media, Pennsylvania 19063-2043 USA

Accurate indications, adverse reactions and dosage schedules for drugs are provided in this book, but it is possible that they may change. The reader is urged to review the package information data of the manufacturers of the medications mentioned.

Printed in the United States of America

Fourth Edition, 1992

Library of Congress Cataloging-in-Publication Data

Chandra, Ramesh, 1938–
  Nuclear medicine physics : the basics / Ramesh Chandra. — 5th ed.
    p.   cm.
  Rev. ed. of: Introductory physics of nuclear medicine. 4th ed. 1992.
  Includes bibliographical references and index.
  ISBN 0-683-30092-X
  1. Medical physics.   2. Nuclear medicine.   3. Radioisotopes.   I. Chandra, Ramesh,
1938–   Introductory physics of nuclear medicine.   II. Title.
    [DNLM: 1. Nuclear Medicine.   2. Health Physics.   3. Radioisotopes.
  WN 110 C457n 1998]
  R895.C47   1998
  616.07′575—dc21
  DNLM/DLC
  for Library of Congress   97-15681
                                                        CIP

The publishers have made every effort to trace the copyright holders for borrowed material. If they have inadvertently overlooked any, they will be pleased to make the necessary arrangements at the first opportunity.

To purchase additional copies of this book, call our customer service department at **(800) 638-0672** or fax orders to **(800) 447-8438**. For other book services, including chapter reprints and large quantity sales, ask for the Special Sales department.

Canadian customers should call **(800) 268-4178**, or fax **(905) 470-6780**. For all other calls originating outside of the United States, please call **(410) 528-4223** or fax us at **(410) 528-8550**.

Visit *Williams & Wilkins* on the Internet: http://www.wwilkins.com or contact our customer service department at **custserv@wwilkins.com**. Williams & Wilkins customer service representatives are available from 8:30 am to 6:00 pm, EST, Monday through Friday, for telephone access.

97 98 99 00 01
1 2 3 4 5 6 7 8 9 10

To my wife, Mithilesh,
my son, Anurag,
and my daughter, Ritu

Preface

The reception of the last edition of this book by resident physicians in radiology and nuclear medicine and by students of nuclear medicine technology has shown a continued need for an introductory book on physics and related basic sciences of nuclear medicine. Therefore, the purpose, the audience, and the level of subject matter remain the same as in previous editions. I quote,

"This book is primarily addressed to resident physicians in nuclear medicine as well as residents in radiology, pathology, and internal medicine who wish to acquire some knowledge of nuclear medicine. Nuclear medicine technicians wishing to advance in their field should also find this book useful.

I have tried to write in a simple and concise manner, including not only essential details but also many examples and problems taken from the routine practice of nuclear medicine. Basic principles and underlying concepts are explained. Mathematical equations or in some cases their derivations have been included only when it was felt their inclusion would help the reader and when it was essential for the proper development of the subject matter. However, the reader is warned that this is not an introductory book of physics, and, therefore, familiarity on his or her part with the elementary concepts of physics, such as units, energy, force, electricity, and light, is assumed by the author."

Keeping the level and spirit of the earlier editions intact, the following major changes have been made in this edition:

1. Seven of 16 chapters (5, 7, 8, 11, 14, 15, and 16) have been thoroughly revised. Besides reorganization of the material, new figures, tables, and text have been added. The enlarged material includes the new radiopharmaceuticals, an updated table of radiation doses from routine nuclear medicine procedures, the new developments in scintillation camera and SPECT, and the recent changes in the rules and regulations governing the usage of radionuclides. Methodology of comparison of radiation risks from various sources of exposure in general and from medical procedures in particular has also been introduced.

2. There are two new appendices—Appendix D: Radionuclides of Interest in Nuclear Medicine; and Appendix E: Organ Masses of a Standard Man.

3. The remaining chapters contain minor changes to add new information or clarify the text.

4. There is a new section at the end of each chapter, "Key Points," describing the important ideas, concepts, and facts discussed in the chapter.

5. The questions, designed to emphasize the salient features and concepts presented in each chapter and to enrich the learning experience of the student by making him or her think and analyze the problem before arriving at the solution, have been enhanced. Answers to the problems have also been provided.

6. Use of both SI and CGS units has been continued because their use in clinical practice persists.

I thank all the people who wrote to me either commending the book or pointing out the errors and omissions in previous editions. Both groups helped me in the preparation of this edition: the first group by boosting my morale and the second group by their suggestions. Individually, I thank Dr. D. Pizzarello, who always made himself available for discussions and served as a sounding board for my ideas. Last, but not least, I thank the publisher and the publisher's staff for their help and cooperation in bringing my labor to fruition.

Ramesh Chandra
New York, New York

Contents

Chapter 6
INTERACTION OF HIGH-ENERGY RADIATION WITH MATTER   50

Chapter 15
BIOLOGICAL EFFECTS OF RADIATION AND RISK EVALUATION
FROM RADIATION EXPOSURE 141

From a physicist's point of view, nature consists mainly of matter and the forces governing the behavior of matter. This chapter reviews briefly some aspects of the atomic structure of matter that are essential for the understanding of subsequent subject matter.

MATTER, ELEMENTS, AND ATOMS

All matter is composed of a limited number of elements (105 identified so far) that in turn are made of atoms. An atom is the smallest part of an element that retains all the chemical properties of that element in bulk. In general, atoms are electrically neutral; that is, they do not show any electric charge. However, atoms are not indivisible as once was thought but are composed of three elementary particles: electrons, protons, and neutrons.

An electron is a tiny particle that possesses a negative charge of 1.6×10^{-19} coulomb (unit of charge) and a mass of 0.9109×10^{-27} g. A proton is a particle with a positive charge equal in amount to that of an electron. A neutron does not have any electric charge and weighs slightly more than a proton. Protons and neutrons have masses of 1.6726×10^{-24} and 1.6747×10^{-24} g, respectively; hence, they are about 2000 times heavier than an electron.

SIMPLIFIED STRUCTURE OF AN ATOM

An atom is generally neutral because it contains the same number of electrons and protons. The number of protons in an atom is also known as the atomic number Z. It specifies the position of that element in the periodic table and therefore specifies its chemical identity. The electrons, protons, and neutrons in an atom are arranged in a planetary structure in which the protons and neutrons (the sun) are located at the center and the electrons (planets) are revolving over the surface of spherical shells (or orbits) of different radii. The center in which the protons and neutrons are located is known as the nucleus and is similar to a packed sphere. The size of atoms of different elements varies greatly but is in the range of 1 to 2×10^{-8} cm. The nucleus is small in comparison to the atom (i.e., about 10^5 times smaller or 10^{-13} cm in size).

The attractive coulomb (electrical) force between the positively charged nucleus (due to the protons) and the negatively charged electrons provides stability to the electrons revolving in the spherical shells. The first shell (having the smallest radius) is known as the K shell, the second shell as L, the third shell as M, and so on. There is a limit to the number of electrons that can occupy a given shell. The K shell can be occupied by a maximum of 2 electrons, the L shell by a maximum of 8 electrons, the M shell by a maximum of 18 electrons, and the N shell by a maximum of 32 electrons. However, the outermost shell in a given atom cannot be occupied by more than eight electrons. In a simple atom like hydrogen, there is only one electron that under normal circumstances occupies the K shell. In a complex atom like iodine, there are 53 electrons that are arranged in the K, L, M, N, and O orbits in numbers of 2, 8, 18, 18, and 7, respectively. The arrangement of electrons in various shells for hydrogen and three other typical atoms is shown in Figure 1.1. This is a simplified description of the atomic structure that, in reality, is more complex as each shell is further divided into subshells. For our purpose, however, it is more than sufficient.

MOLECULES

Molecules are formed by the combination of two or more atoms (e.g., a molecule of water, H_2O, is formed by the combination of two hydrogen atoms and one oxygen atom). The combination of atoms is accomplished through the interaction of electrons (also known as valent electrons) in the outermost orbits of the atom. Valent electrons participate in the formation of the molecules in several ways—for example, in ionic binding, covalent binding, and hydrogen binding. In theory, most chemical reactions and chemical properties of atoms or molecules can

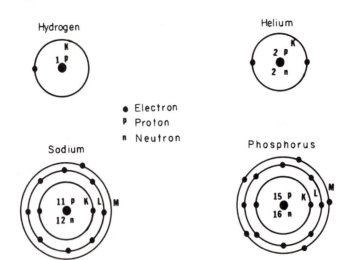

Figure 1.1.   Simplified atomic structure of four elements in their ground state.

be explained on the basis of the interaction of the valent electrons.

BINDING ENERGY, IONIZATION, AND EXCITATION

Each electron in a given shell is bound to the nucleus with a fixed amount of energy. Therefore, if one wishes to remove an electron from a particular shell to make it free and no longer associated with that atom, energy will have to be provided to the electron from outside the atom. The minimum amount of the energy necessary to free an electron from an atom is known as the binding energy of the electron in that atom. The unit in which energy is measured on the atomic scale is known as an electron volt (eV), which is the energy acquired by an electron accelerated through 1 V of potential difference. The electrons in the K shell are the most tightly bound electrons in an atom and therefore require the most energy to be removed from the atom (removal of an electron from an atom is called ionization). Electrons in the outermost shell, on the other hand, are the least tightly bound electrons and therefore require the least amount of energy for their removal from the atom. The binding energy of electrons in various shells increases rapidly with the atomic number Z. Table 1.1 lists the K- and L-shell average binding energies of electrons in the atoms of various elements.

Under normal conditions, electrons occupy the lowest possible shells (those closest to the nucleus) consistent with the maximum number of electrons by which a given shell can be occupied. However, electrons can be made to move into higher shells (unoccupied shells) temporarily by the absorption of energy. This absorption can take place in various ways—for example, by heating a substance, by subjecting matter to high electric fields, by passage of a charged particle through matter, or even by a high mechanical impact. When an electron absorbs sufficient energy for its removal from the atom, the process is called ionization and the remaining atom, an ion. When the electron absorbs amounts of en-

Table 1.1.   Average Binding Energies of K- and L-Shell Electrons in Various Elements

Element	Atomic Number Z	Average Binding Energy (keV)	
		K Shell	L Shell
H	1	0.014	—
C	6	0.28	0.007
O	8	0.53	0.024
P	15	2.15	0.19
S	16	2.47	0.23
Fe	26	7.11	0.85
Zn	30	9.66	1.19
Br	35	13.47	1.78
Ag	47	25.51	3.81
I	53	33.17	5.19
Tm	69	59.40	10.12
W	74	69.52	12.10
Pb	82	88.00	15.86

ergy that are just sufficient to move it into a higher unoccupied shell, the process is known as excitation and the atom as an excited atom. Excited atoms are, in general, unstable and acquire their normal configuration by emitting electromagnetic radiation (light, ultraviolet light or x-rays), generally within 10^{-9} seconds.

For example, let us consider a sodium atom, which has an atomic number of 11 and therefore 11 electrons and 11 protons. The electrons are arranged in K, L, and M shells in numbers of two, eight, and one, respectively. The energies of these electrons in the K, L, and M shells are approximately -1072, -63, and -1 eV, respectively. To remove an electron from the K shell of a sodium atom, it is necessary to provide an amount of energy equal to 1072 eV, whereas from the M shell only 1 eV of energy is necessary. An electron from the L shell can move to the M shell by absorbing 62 eV of energy, thereby producing an excited atom of sodium. When this excited atom decays (i.e., when the electron jumps back into the L shell), an electromagnetic radiation of 62 eV will be emitted.

It should be pointed out here that in the case of electrons, the zero of energy scale, by convention, is chosen to be the state when the electron is just free and not bound to the atom. As a result, when an electron is bound in the atom, its energy is represented as negative and when an electron is free and moving (i.e., possesses kinetic energy), its energy is represented as positive. This convention is different from the one used in the case of nucleus discussed in the next chapter (p. 13).

FORCES OR FIELDS

Force is a general term related to the interaction of various constituents of matter. At present, four kinds of forces (or fields) are known: gravitational, weak, electromagnetic, and strong. Gravitational forces are produced as a result of the mass of matter and play a significant role in holding our solar system intact, but they are negligible between atoms and molecules. Weak forces play a significant part in nuclear transformation, which is described in Chapter 2. Electromagnetic forces play a dominant role in our daily life, because they hold the atom together and are responsible for interactions between atoms, molecules, biomolecules, and so on. Strong forces are the forces that hold a nucleus together and act between proton–

proton, proton–neutron, and neutron–neutron. The relative strengths of these forces are listed below.

Type of Force	Strength
Strong	1
Electromagnetic	10^{-2}
Weak	10^{-13}
Gravitational	10^{-39}

Electromagnetic Forces

Electromagnetic forces or fields are produced by charged particles. During interaction between charged particles, quite often energy is emitted as electromagnetic radiation. Electromagnetic radiation can propagate either as waves or as particles. When electromagnetic radiation behaves like particles, these particles are called photons. A photon does not have any rest mass or charge. It is a packet of energy that interacts with matter in a specified manner or according to the laws of electromagnetic forces. The dual nature of radiation, which is now an established fact, is true of matter (i.e., electrons) as well. Electromagnetic radiation is characterized by its energy or wavelength only. Electromagnetic radiation of varying energies is known by different names (Fig. 1.2). The energy of electromagnetic radiation is related to the wavelength by a simple relationship:

$$E = \frac{hc}{\lambda}$$

where h is Planck's constant, c is the velocity of light or electromagnetic radiation, and λ is the wavelength. The above relationship is further reduced if one measures energy in keV and the wavelength in angstroms ($\text{Å} = 10^{-8}$ cm):

$$E \text{ (keV)} = \frac{12.4}{\lambda}$$

CHARACTERISTIC X-RAYS AND AUGER ELECTRONS

As can be seen from Figure 1.2, x-rays are part of the electromagnetic radiation spectrum. Electromagnetic radiations with energies of approximately 100 eV or more are called x-rays. X-rays are primarily distinguished from other forms of electromagnetic radiation by their ability to produce ionization in matter and to pene-

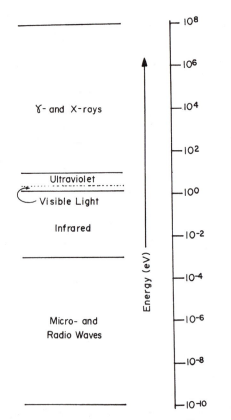

Figure 1.2. Spectrum of electromagnetic waves. Electromagnetic waves of different energies are known by various names. For example, x- or γ-waves are electromagnetic waves with energies higher than 100 eV.

trate substances. Characteristic x-rays are produced by the transition of electrons from outer to inner orbits of atoms (the K or L shell in most cases). The inner orbits of an atom under normal circumstances are fully occupied; therefore, to cause the transition of an electron from an outer to an inner orbit, it is necessary to create a vacancy or hole in the inner orbit. This can be accomplished in various ways. The well-known example is an x-ray tube, where high-energy electrons sometimes collide with the inner-shell electrons, knocking them out of the target atoms and thus creating a vacancy in the inner shells of the target atoms. Other examples of vacancy creation in inner shells are discussed in Chapter 2.

Once a vacancy is created in the inner shell of an atom, an electron from the outer shell falls to fill this hole. The difference between the potential energies of the two shells involved in the transition is emitted as electromagnetic radiation. This is called a characteristic x-ray of the atom if the energy emitted is approximately 100

eV or more. If the vacancy was in the K shell, the x-rays emitted are known as K x-rays; if the vacancy was in the L shell, they are known as L x-rays. Because the energy of a characteristic x-ray emitted by an atom is unique, it is possible to identify an atom (and therefore an element) by the energy of its characteristic x-rays.

Let us consider the example of a sodium atom where electrons in the K, L, and M shells have -1072, -63, and -1 eV of energies, respectively. Now if a vacancy is created in the K shell of this atom, it will be filled by one of the L- or M-shell electrons. Let us assume it is filled by the L-shell electron. The L-shell electron, which originally had an energy of -63 eV, now in the K shell has only -1072 eV energy. The balance of this energy, $e_L - e_K = [-63 - (-1072)] = 1009$ eV, will be emitted as a characteristic K x-ray and its energy is unique for sodium atom.

An alternate process to characteristic x-ray emission is the emission of Auger electrons (named in honor of their discoverer, P. Auger). In this process, the vacancy in the K shell is filled by an electron from the L or M shells; however, the balance of energy that would have been emitted as an x-ray is taken by another electron from the L or M shell. Thus, in Auger-electron emission, two electrons are removed from L and/or M shells: one fills the vacancy in K shell, and the other is emitted from the atom with the balance of energy. The atom is now doubly ionized. A similar process may occur if the vacancy is in the L or M shell. The Auger process occurs most frequently in elements with low atomic numbers ($Z < 24$, e.g., C, N, O, Al, Ca), whereas x-ray emission is characteristic of elements with high atomic numbers ($Z > 45$, e.g., I, Cs, W, Pb). These two processes, characteristic x-ray emission and Auger-electron emission, are graphically depicted in Figure 1.3.

INTERCHANGEABILITY OF MASS AND ENERGY

In 1905, Einstein derived an expression on theoretical grounds that showed the interconvertibility of mass and energy. With subsequent advances in experimental atomic and nuclear physics, his assertion proved to be correct. The expression that relates mass and energy is simply

$$E = mc^2$$

where E is the energy, m is the mass, and c is the

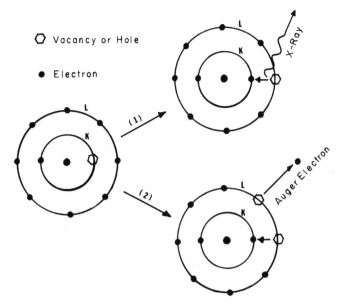

Figure 1.3. X-ray emission and Auger-electron emission. When there is a vacancy (or hole) in the K shell of an atom, one of two processes may occur: either an electron from the L shell (or higher shells) fills the vacancy in the K shell and the balance of energy between the K and L shells is emitted as a characteristic x-ray, or one of the electrons from the L shell fills the vacancy in the K shell and the balance of energy is taken by another electron in the L shell (or higher shell), which is then emitted as an Auger electron.

velocity of light. Mass on an atomic or nuclear scale is measured in atomic mass units (amu), defined as $\frac{1}{12}$ of the mass of a carbon atom. From Einstein's equation for mass and energy conversion, 1 amu is equivalent to 931 MeV of energy. The masses in amu and their equivalent energy in MeV for an electron, proton, and neutron are given in Table 1.2.

Table 1.2. Mass and Energy Equivalence for Electrons, Protons, and Neutrons

Particle	Mass (amu)	Mass Energy (MeV)
e	0.000549	0.511
p	1.00728	938.28
n	1.00867	939.57

Key Points

1. Matter is made of a relatively small number of elements. An atom is the smallest chemical unit of an element.

2. An atom is made of elementary particles, electrons, protons, and neutrons. Electrons revolve in fixed orbits, K, L, M, and so on, around the nucleus that contains both protons and neutrons. Electrons are bound in orbits with fixed amount of energies, called binding energy. Number of electrons equals number of protons, Z (atomic number), in a neutral atom.

3. Electrons can move to higher orbits by ab-sorption of energy in discrete amounts, thus producing excited atoms. Electrons can be completely removed from an atom by absorption of energies that exceed the binding energies of the electrons, causing the atom to be ionized.

4. Excited atoms release their energy in the form of electromagnetic radiation.

5. Elementary particles interact with each other through four types of forces of which electromagnetic force is the dominant force between electrons and the nucleus. It provides stability to electrons revolving in the orbits.

6. Electromagnetic force manifests itself as waves or particles called photons. Photons of different energies are known by different names, such as x- or γ-rays, ultraviolet light, visible light, infrared light, microwaves and radio waves. Energy of a photon is related to its frequency or wavelength by the following expression: $E = hc/\lambda$.

7. Mass and energy are interchangeable and are related through Einstein's equation, $E = mc^2$.

Questions

1. Find the energies of radiations emitted from the atoms of (a) iodine and (b) lead when there is a vacancy in the K shell of these atoms (use Table 1.1).

2. Determine the minimum energy needed to create a vacancy in (a) the K shells of P, Fe, and Tm atoms and (b) the L shells of Zn, I, and Pb atoms.

3. What are the wavelengths of the 10, 100, and 1000 keV x-rays?

4. If the rest mass of an electron is converted into electromagnetic energy, what is the energy of this radiation? What is its name?

5. If the mass difference between a neutron and a proton can be converted into electrons, what is the maximum number of electrons produced?

2   Nuclides and Radioactive Processes

In the previous chapter, I discussed the structure of the atom and pointed out the importance of electrons and their interaction. In this chapter, I discuss the properties of the nucleus (the central core of an atom) and the radioactive processes that are strictly nuclear phenomena.

NUCLIDES AND THEIR CLASSIFICATION

As in the case of an atom, different types of atoms are called elements; in the case of a nucleus, different types of nuclei are termed nuclides. An element is characterized by its atomic number (Z) alone, whereas a nuclide is characterized by its mass number (A) and by its atomic number (Z). The mass number (A) of a nuclide is the sum of the number of its protons (Z) and neutrons (N), that is, $A = Z + N$.

As an example, $^{131}_{53}I$, a nuclide of iodine, contains 53 protons and 78 neutrons, which add up to 131, the mass number of this nuclide. A general notation for a nuclide is $^A_Z X$, where A and Z are, respectively, the mass number and atomic number of the nuclide and X is the element to which this nuclide belongs.

Nuclides are classified according to their mass number, neutron number, and atomic (proton) number. Nuclides having the same *atomic mass* are called *isobars* (e.g., $^{131}_{53}I$ and $^{131}_{54}Xe$; both of these nuclides have the same mass number, 131). Nuclides having the same number of *protons* are called *isotopes* (e.g., $^{12}_6C$ and $^{13}_6C$). Because they contain the same number of protons and therefore have the same atomic number, isotopes always belong to the same element. Nuclides having the same number of *neutrons* are called *isotones* (e.g., $^{13}_7N$ and $^{14}_8O$; both of these nuclides contain six neutrons). As an aid to memory, a pair of corresponding letters in each definition are italicized.

same number of *protons*	iso*to*pes
same *atomic* mass	iso*ba*rs
same number of *neutrons*	iso*tones*

NUCLEAR STRUCTURE AND EXCITED STATES OF A NUCLIDE

How are neutrons and protons (a common name for the two combined is nucleon) arranged inside the nucleus? We have only a partial answer to this question so far. Our understanding of the structure of a nucleus as compared with the structure of an atom (i.e., arrangement of electrons in various shells and their interactions) is quite limited. It is postulated—with a wealth of supportive experimental data—that nucleons are arranged in spherical shells inside the nucleus in a manner similar to that of electrons in an atom. Not much is known, however, of the manner in which nucleons are stacked in these shells or about the transitions of nucleons between different shells. What is known and is important for the present discussion is that nucleons, like electrons in an atom, can also be excited to higher unoccupied shells by absorption of energy from outside the nucleus. The lowest possible arrangement of nucleons in the nucleus is known as the ground state of a nuclide. The higher shells are commonly referred to as energy levels or excited states. Again, similar to electrons in an atom, nucleons in a nucleus are also bound with different binding energies. The binding energy of a nucleon (amount of energy needed to pull it out of the nucleus) varies from nuclide to nuclide. However, the average binding energy of nucleons for most nuclides is in the range of 5 to 8 MeV. This is about 1000 times higher (MeV rather than keV) than the average binding energies of electrons in atoms. Therefore, it is hard to remove a proton or neutron from a nucleus. It requires transfer of a large amount of energy from outside that is, in general, only possible in nuclear reactors, accelerators, or cyclotrons.

The excited states of a nuclide, in general, are of a short duration ($< 10^{-11}$ seconds) and decay to the ground state or lower energy states by emission of high-energy radiation in a manner similar to that of the excited states of an atom, which decay to the ground state of an atom by emitting light or x-rays.

Excited states have the same mass number, same atomic number, and the same number of neutrons as the ground state and therefore are called isomers (i.e., an isomer is an excited state of a nuclide). Note that the letter e has been italicized twice in the above definition, again as an aid to memory. The isomer of a nuclide is generally distinguished from its ground state by placing an asterisk after the symbol of the nuclide (e.g., $^{12}_{6}C^*$ is an excited state of $^{12}_{6}C$). In a few cases, however, the lifetime of the excited state of a nuclide can be very long (seconds, minutes, or even years). When this occurs, the excited state is called a metastable state. Well-known examples of nuclides having metastable states are ^{99m}Tc and ^{113m}In. The letter "m" after the mass number in these two nuclides stands for metastable state and distinguishes them from their respective ground states of ^{99}Tc and ^{113}In.

RADIONUCLIDES AND STABILITY OF NUCLIDES

Even in their ground state, many nuclides are unstable. These unstable nuclides are called radionuclides. Radionuclides try to become stable by emitting electromagnetic radiation or charged particles. Electromagnetic radiation or charged particle emission is called radioactive decay. What makes a nuclide stable or radioactive? Two kinds of forces, strong and electromagnetic, determine the stability of a nuclide. The strong forces act between a pair of nucleons (e.g., proton–proton, proton–neutron, or neutron–neutron). They are attractive and act only when the distance between the two nucleons is very small. Electromagnetic forces act between protons only (because there is no charge on neutrons) and are repulsive (similar charges repel each other). The balance between these two forces—one attractive, the other repulsive—determines the stability of a nuclide. Whenever the balance between these two forces is disturbed, the nuclide becomes unstable and therefore radioactive. There are approximately 259 stable nuclides found in nature. If one plots the number of neutrons (N) contained as a function of the number of protons (Z) in a nuclide for all stable nuclides, a curve as shown in Figure 2.1 results. This curve initially starts as a straight line and then slowly bends toward the neutron number (N) for higher atomic numbers. From this curve it can be seen that for

Figure 2.1. Plot of the number of neutrons as a function of number of protons (atomic number) for stable nuclides. In the low-atomic-number elements, the number of protons is roughly equal to the number of neutrons, but in the higher-atomic-number elements, more neutrons are needed than protons for stability. Radionuclides lie on either side of the stability curve.

a lighter nuclide (A < 50), the number of protons in stable nuclides is equal to the number of neutrons; for example, $^{16}_{8}O$, a stable oxygen nuclide, contains eight neutrons and eight protons. For heavier nuclides (A > 100), however, the number of neutrons needed for the stability of a nuclide is much more than the number of protons; for example, $^{127}_{53}I$, a stable iodine nuclide, contains 53 protons and 74 neutrons. The region on either side of the curve in Figure 2.1 is called the domain of radionuclides. If a radionuclide lies in the upper region, it contains an excess number of neutrons that cause the unstability of the radionuclide. On the other hand, if the radionuclide lies in the lower region, it is the excess of protons that makes the nuclide unstable.

RADIOACTIVE SERIES OR CHAIN

A radionuclide tries to attain stability through radioactive decay. The stability may be achieved either by direct (single-step) decay to a stable nuclide or by decaying to several radionuclides in multiple steps and, finally, to a stable nuclide.

For example, $^{131}_{53}$I directly decays to a stable nuclide $^{131}_{54}$Xe. On the other hand, $^{226}_{88}$Ra first decays to $^{222}_{86}$Rn, which decays to $^{218}_{84}$Po. . . , and finally to $^{210}_{82}$Pb, a stable nuclide. The complete series for this is given below (the arrows denote the sequence of decay).

$$^{226}_{88}\text{Ra} \rightarrow\, ^{222}_{86}\text{Rn} \rightarrow\, ^{218}_{84}\text{Po} \rightarrow\, ^{214}_{82}\text{Pb} \rightarrow\, ^{214}_{83}\text{Bi} \rightarrow\,$$
$$^{214}_{84}\text{Po} \rightarrow\, ^{210}_{82}\text{Pb (stable nuclide)}$$

This latter process is often referred to as a radioactive series or chain. Well-known examples of a radioactive series in nuclear medicine are the decay of ^{99}Mo and ^{113}Sn, which go through the following sequences:

$$^{99}\text{Mo} \rightarrow\, ^{99m}\text{Tc} \rightarrow\, ^{99}\text{Tc} \rightarrow\, ^{99}\text{Ru (stable)}$$
$$^{113}\text{Sn} \rightarrow\, ^{113m}\text{In} \rightarrow\, ^{113}\text{In (stable)}$$

RADIOACTIVE PROCESSES AND CONSERVATION LAWS

The three processes through which a radionuclide tries to attain stability are called alpha, beta, and gamma decay. These names were given because at the time of the discovery of these processes their exact nature was not known. Three important conservation laws are pertinent here because they always hold true in radioactive processes or nuclear transformations. These are the law of conservation of energy, the law of conservation of mass number, and the law of conservation of electric charge.

The law of conservation of energy states that the total energy (mass energy + kinetic energy + energy in any other form, e.g., a photon) remains unchanged during a radioactive process or nuclear transformation. The law of conservation of mass number states that the sum of mass numbers remains unchanged in radioactive or nuclear processes. The mass number of a neutron or proton is assumed to be one and that of an electron zero. Similarly, the law of conservation of electric charge states that the total charge during a radioactive process or nuclear transformation remains unchanged.

Alpha Decay

In alpha decay, a radionuclide emits a heavy, charged particle called an α particle. An α particle is four times heavier than a proton or neutron and carries an electric charge that is twice that of a proton. In fact, an α particle is a stable nuclide

with atomic mass number A = 4 and atomic number Z = 2. This happens to be the nucleus of a helium atom.

From the conservation laws of the mass number and electric charge, it follows that during alpha decay the mass number and the atomic number of the resulting nuclide (also known as the daughter nuclide) will be reduced by 4 and 2, respectively. Alpha decay can be expressed by the following equation:

$$^A_Z\text{X} = \,^{(A-4)}_{(Z-2)}\text{Y} + \,^4_2\text{He (}\alpha\text{ particle)}$$

Notice that the mass number and the electric charge (in this case the sum of atomic numbers) on both sides of the equation are the same. An example of alpha decay is the decay of radium-226 to radon-222:

$$^{226}_{88}\text{Ra} = \,^{222}_{86}\text{Rn} + \alpha$$

EXAMPLE:

$^{222}_{86}$Rn is a radionuclide that decays through alpha decay. Determine the nature of its daughter nuclide. Because $^{222}_{86}$Rn decays through the alpha decay process, the mass number of the daughter nuclide will be 4 less than that of the parent, that is, $222 - 4 = 218$. Similarly, the atomic number will be reduced by 2, that is, $86 - 2 = 84$. Therefore, the daughter nuclide has a mass number 218 and its atomic number is 84. According to the periodic table, the atomic number 84 belongs to the element Po. Therefore, the daughter nuclide is $^{218}_{84}$Po.

Radon-222 is a radioactive gas that escapes into the environment from the rocks or soil containing radium-226. A small amount of radium is present everywhere. Such amounts are generally no more than a nuisance that increases the background radiation slightly. However, a combination of relatively large concentrations of radium in the soil and rocks and poor circulation in a house can sometimes produce hazardous concentrations of radon in the house, which have to be dealt with effectively for the safety of the occupants.

Two salient facts concerning alpha decay to remember are: it occurs mostly with radionuclides whose atomic mass number A is greater than 150 and the kinetic energy of the emitted α particle is fixed and discrete for a given decay. In the above example of $^{226}_{88}$Ra alpha decay, the kinetic energy of the α particle emitted is 4.780 MeV.

Beta Decay

During this transformation, a neutron or a proton inside the nucleus of a radionuclide is converted to a proton or a neutron, respectively. When a proton is converted into a neutron, the positive charge inside the nucleus decreases by one, reducing the repulsive forces between protons. On the other hand, when a neutron is converted into a proton, the positive charge inside the nucleus increases by one, and therefore the repulsive forces between protons are increased. The result of the decrease or increase in the repulsive force within the nucleus is to balance the two forces (electromagnetic and strong) in an attempt to stabilize the nuclide (see Radionuclides and Stability of Nuclides, p. 8).

The conversion of a neutron into a proton or of a proton into a neutron is controlled by weak (as opposed to strong, electromagnetic, and gravitational) forces (see Chapter 1). The exact nature of weak forces is not known and is not pertinent to our discussion of beta decay. Beta decay occurs through one of the following processes: β^- emission or electron emission, β^+ emission or positron emission, or electron capture.

β^- EMISSION

In this process, a neutron inside the radionuclide is converted into a proton and the excess energy is released as a pair of particles, an electron and an antineutrino ($\overline{\nu}$). As such, there are no electrons or antineutrinos inside the nucleus. These are created from excess energy at the instant of radioactive decay. An antineutrino is a particle that has no rest mass and no electric charge ($Z = 0$). It rarely interacts with matter and therefore is of no biological significance. Its existence was postulated so that the law of energy conservation would not be violated. However, its existence has now been confirmed experimentally. β^- decay can be expressed as

$$_Z^A X = {}_{Z+1}^A Y + e^- + \overline{\nu}$$

Note that both the mass number and the electric charge are conserved. Some well-known examples of β^- decay are $_1^3 H$, $_6^{14} C$, and $_{15}^{32} P$, which can be expressed as follows:

$$_1^3 H = {}_2^3 He + e^- + \overline{\nu}$$
$$_6^{14} C = {}_7^{14} N + e^- + \overline{\nu}$$
$$_{15}^{32} P = {}_{16}^{32} S + e^- + \overline{\nu}$$

As can be seen, during β^- decay the mass number (A) remains unchanged and the atomic number (Z) is increased by one. The kinetic energy of the emitted electron is not fixed because the total available energy in the decay (difference between the mass energy of the parent radionuclide and the daughter nuclide) has to be shared between the electron and the antineutrino.

In the above example, the difference between the mass energies of $_1^3 H$ and $_2^3 He$, $_6^{14} C$ and $_7^{14} N$, and $_{15}^{32} P$ and $_{16}^{32} S$ during decay is shared by the electron and the antineutrino. The sharing of the available energy is random; therefore, the electrons are emitted with varying amounts of kinetic energy (known as the β^- spectrum) ranging from 0 to a maximum of E_β max. E_β max is the total available energy in the case of a particular β^- decay. In the above examples E_β max for ^3H decay is 0.018 MeV; for ^{14}C decay it is 0.156 MeV; for ^{32}P decay it is 1.71 MeV. The probability of an electron emission with a given kinetic energy E_β, $P(E_\beta)$, varies greatly with the kinetic energy E_β. The variation of $P(E_\beta)$ with E_β (i.e., β^- spectrum) is shown in Figure 2.2 for a typical β^- decay.

In calculations of radiation dose to a patient with β^--emitting radionuclides, one is interested in the average energy, $\overline{E}_\beta$, of the electrons. The computation of $\overline{E}_\beta$ depends on knowledge of the exact shape of β spectrum. However, as a rule of

Figure 2.2. A typical β-ray spectrum. In beta decay, electrons (or positrons) are emitted with varying energies up to a maximum E_β max. A β spectrum gives the probability of emission of an electron with a given energy E_β.

thumb, in cases where high accuracy is not desired, $\overline{E}_\beta$ can be obtained by dividing E_β max by 3 (i.e., $\overline{E}_\beta = E_\beta$ max/3). Generally, E_β max, and usually $\overline{E}_\beta$, is listed in the table of nuclides.

β⁺ OR POSITRON EMISSION

In this process, a proton inside the nucleus is converted into a neutron and the excess energy is emitted as a pair of particles, in this case a positron and a neutrino. (Neutrinos and antineutrinos can be considered identical for our purposes.) A positron is an electron with a unit-positive instead of a unit-negative charge. It has the same mass as an electron and interacts with matter in a manner similar to that of an electron. Positron decay can be expressed as

$$^A_Z X = {}_{Z-1}^A Y + e^+ + \nu$$

This equation is consistent with the laws of conservation of mass number and electric charge. However, for the total energy to be conserved, the mass of the nuclide X should be greater than the mass of the Y nuclide by at least 1.02 MeV (2 × mass of an electron). This is because the mass of a nuclide includes in it the mass of the nucleus and the electrons associated with it. Therefore, the mass of the X nuclide contains the mass of Z electrons, whereas the mass of the Y nuclide contains the mass of only Z − 1 electrons. Also an e⁺ is created from the nuclear energy of X nuclide. Hence, the mass of the X nuclide has to be greater than 2 × the mass of an electron plus the mass of Y nuclide. Some examples of positron emission are

$$^{11}_6 C = {}^{11}_5 B + e^+ + \nu$$
$$^{15}_8 O = {}^{15}_7 N + e^+ + \nu$$
$$^{18}_9 F = {}^{18}_8 O + e^+ + \nu$$

Note that during β⁺ emission, the mass number does not change, but the atomic number is decreased by one. In β⁺ emission, too, the energy of the emitted positron varies from 0 to maximum E_β max, which is known as β⁺ spectrum. The exact computation of the average β⁺ energy, $\overline{E}_\beta{}^+$, in this case, too, is quite involved. As an approximation one can determine $\overline{E}_\beta{}^+$ again by dividing the $E_\beta{}^+$ max by three.

ELECTRON CAPTURE

In this process, a proton inside the nucleus is converted into a neutron by capturing an electron from one of the atomic shells (e.g., K, L, or M). No electron or positron but only a neutrino is emitted. The capture of an electron from the K shell of the atom is known as K capture; capture of an electron from the L shell is known as L capture and so on. Electron capture is one of the few instances (another will be encountered in the case of gamma decay) in which a nucleus interacts directly with the orbital (K, L shells, etc.) electrons of an atom. Once an electron is captured from the K, L, or M shell, a vacancy is created in the inner shell of an atom. This vacancy is subsequently filled by electrons from higher shells with simultaneous emission of a characteristic x-ray or Auger electron (see Chapter 1). The probability of a capture from the K shell is generally much higher than that from the L or M shell. Electron capture is expressed as

$$^A_Z X + e^- \text{ (orbital)} = {}_{Z-1}^A Y + \nu$$

This is also consistent with the laws of conservation of mass number and electric charge. Common examples of electron capture are

$$^{51}_{24} Cr + e^- \text{ (orbital)} = {}^{51}_{23} V + \nu$$
$$^{131}_{55} Cs + e^- \text{ (orbital)} = {}^{131}_{54} Xe + \nu$$

Note that during electron capture, as in positron emission, the mass number does not change but the atomic number is reduced by one.

During all three processes of beta decay, the mass number A remains unchanged. For this reason, beta decay is quite often referred to as an isobaric transition.

Gamma Decay or Isomeric Transition

It has already been explained that a nucleus can be excited by the absorption of energy to an excited state (isomer). Isomers in general are of very short duration except in cases of metastable states. The decay of an excited state to a lower energy or ground state is known as isomeric transition (as opposed to isobaric transition in the case of beta decay) and proceeds through either of two processes: an emission of a high-energy photon, or internal conversion. These are graphically shown in Figure 2.3.

HIGH-ENERGY PHOTON EMISSION

In this process, the excess energy of an isomer is released in the form of a high-energy photon

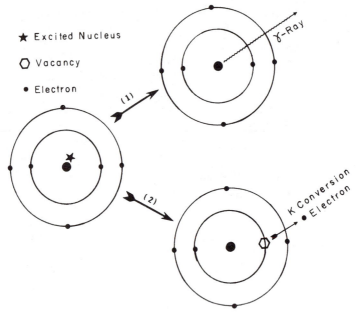

Figure 2.3.   Isomeric transition. An excited nucleus in isomeric transition can release its energy in two ways: by the emission of γ-ray (photon) or by the transfer of its energy directly to an orbital electron, generally in the K shell. The electron acquiring the energy is ejected from the atom and is known as the conversion electron. The vacancy thus created in the inner shell of the atom is subsequently filled in the manner discussed in Chapter 1.

known as a γ-ray. A γ-ray is an electromagnetic radiation with high energy (>100 eV; see Chapter 1). A γ-ray and an x-ray of the same energy cannot be distinguished from each other because both interact with matter in exactly the same manner. The only difference between the two is that of origin. Energy emitted from the nucleus as a high-energy photon is known as a γ-ray; energy emitted by an atom (i.e., transition of electrons in atomic shells) as a high-energy photon is called an x-ray. This difference in nomenclature of a high-energy photon is of no practical significance in nuclear medicine.

INTERNAL CONVERSION

Sometimes a nuclide in an excited state, instead of emitting a γ-ray, transfers its excess energy directly to an orbital electron (in the K, L, or M shell). This process is called internal conversion and is another example of the direct interaction of a nucleus with the orbital electrons revolving around it. (Electron capture in beta decay, the first example, is described on p. 11.)

Internal conversion is an alternate process to γ-ray emission. A single nucleus will emit either a

γ-ray or an electron. However, in a collection of nuclei, some will emit γ-rays and some conversion electrons. The ratio of the number of electrons to the number of γ-rays emitted by a collection of excited nuclei is called the coefficient of internal conversion (ic) for that excited state:

$$ic = \frac{\text{total number of electrons emitted}}{\text{total number of } \gamma\text{-rays emitted}}$$

When considering only the electrons knocked from the K shell, the above ratio is known as the coefficient of K conversion, ic_K. When considering only the electrons knocked out of the L shell, the above ratio is known as the coefficient of L conversion, ic_L. The total conversion coefficient, then, is the sum of the individual K, L, M conversion coefficients (i.e., ic = $ic_K + ic_L + ic_M$).

As an example, if ic = $\frac{1}{5}$, the emission of a γ-ray is five times more likely than the emission of an electron by internal conversion, or out of six decays, five will be through γ-ray or photon emission, and only one will be through the conversion process. Therefore, if there are 100 decays of excited nuclei, then in $\frac{5}{6} \times 100 \approx 83$ decays a γ-ray will be emitted, and in the remaining 17 decays a conversion electron will be emitted. If the internal conversion coefficient, ic, is 2, then the emission of an electron is twice as likely as the emission of a γ-ray, or out of three decays, one will be through γ-ray emission and two will be through conversion electron emission. Therefore, if there are 100 decays of the excited nuclei, then the number of γ-rays emitted will be $\frac{1}{3} \times 100 \simeq 33$, whereas the number of conversion electrons emitted will be 67. When I discuss later the ideal properties of a radionuclide for nuclear medicine (Chapter 5), it will be seen that radionuclides that do not emit particulate radiation are desirable. Since even in gamma decay, because of internal conversion, electrons can be emitted, it follows that the coefficient of internal conversion should be as small as possible.

The probability of K conversion is generally quite high compared with L and M conversion because of the closeness of the K-shell electrons to the nucleus compared with the L- and M-shell electrons. Also, the probability of internal conversion is higher if the excited state is long-lived (metastable state) and the energy of the excited state is low (<100 keV).

Because in internal conversion an electron is emitted from the inner shell of an atom (K, L, or M), a vacancy is created in that shell. This vacancy is subsequently filled by electrons from higher shells, leading to the emission of an x-ray or Auger electron. The process of vacancy filling in atomic shells is the same as that following K capture in beta decay. As the electrons in each shell (K, L, . . .) of the atom are bound with a certain amount of energy known as binding energy, the conversion electron carries a kinetic energy that is the difference of the energy of the excited state (nucleus) and the binding energy of the electron in a given shell. For example, ^{113m}In, a metastable state with an energy of 393 keV, emits a γ-ray of 393 keV but emits a K conversion electron with a kinetic energy of 393 − 29.7 (B.E. of K electrons in In atom) = 363.3 keV.

DECAY SCHEMES

In this discussion of alpha, beta, and gamma decay, various examples of radioactive processes have been presented. How does one know that a

given radionuclide will decay by the emission of an α particle, β-ray, or γ-ray or by a combination of two or more? Actually, there are no theoretical laws to supply this information. Such data are experimentally determined for each radionuclide and then tabulated in a pictorial form known as a decay scheme. A decay scheme is a collection of experimental information regarding the modes and frequency of decay, process of decay, energy of different radiation emitted, half-life, and other information of interest for a given radionuclide.

In one commonly used approach, decay schemes of isobars (or β transitions) are graphically represented on one page, with radionuclides arranged in order of increasing atomic number from left to right. In this representation, all β⁻-decaying radionuclides decay to the nuclide on their right (↘) and all the K-capture or e⁺-decaying radionuclides to their left (↙ or ↓). A broken arrow is the indication for positron decay. It signifies that the mass of the parent nuclide has to be greater than the mass of the daughter nuclide by at least 1.02 MeV. The excited states of the nuclides are shown as horizontal bars above the ground state. The energy of these states increases from the bottom to the top of the page. Isomeric transitions between two states are shown by vertical lines connecting the two states.

In this instance, as opposed to the energy of electrons in an atom (p. 3), the zero of the energy scale is, by convention, chosen to be the ground state of a nuclide. It is as if the K shell of an atom has been arbitrarily chosen to have zero energy. According to this convention, then, all other shells of the atom (L, M, etc.) will have positive energy. In nuclear convention, then, the energy of the electrons in the K, L, and M shells of a sodium atom will, instead of −1072, −63, and −1 eV, be 0, 1009, and 1071 eV, respectively.

A decay scheme is shown in Figure 2.4 for ^{99}Mo, the parent of ^{99m}Tc that has revolutionized the field of nuclear medicine. Briefly, the decay scheme of ^{99}Mo shows that ^{99}Mo decays 80% of the time to an excited state of ^{99}Tc, which has an energy of 0.142 MeV (a metastable state because of its relatively long life), by emission of a β⁻ particle with E_β max = 1.23 MeV. For 18.5% of the time, the decay proceeds to an-

Figure 2.4.   Decay scheme of ^{99}Mo. ^{99}Mo decays via β emission to the 0.142, 0.513, and 0.922 MeV excited states of ^{99}Tc. These excited states then decay to the ground state by the emission of a number of γ-rays shown above. Less likely transitions have been omitted from the decay scheme. Except for the 0.142 MeV state, which has a half-life of 6 hours, other excited states are short lived.

Table 2.1.   Radiations Emitted in the Decay of ^{99}Mo

Number	Radiation (i)	Frequency of Emission (n_i)	Mean Energy (MeV) ($\bar{E}_i$)
1	β 1	0.185	0.140
2	β 2	0.014	0.298
3	β 3	0.797	0.452
4	γ 1	—	—
5	M conversion electron	0.851	0.002
6	γ 2	0.130	0.041
7	K conversion electron	0.043	0.019
8	γ 3	0.815	0.140
9	K conversion electron	0.085	0.120
10	L conversion electron	0.011	0.138
11	γ 4	—	—
12	γ 5	0.066	0.181
13	γ 6	0.014	0.366
14	γ 7	0.137	0.740
15	γ 8	0.048	0.778
16	X-rays—K(α)	0.094	0.018
17	X-rays—K(β)	0.017	0.021
18	KLL Auger electron	0.022	0.015
19	KLX Auger electron	0.01	0.018
20	LMM Auger electron	1.53	0.002
21	MXY Auger electron	1.20	0.001

Figure 2.5. Decay scheme of ^{99m}Tc: the 6-hour half-life isomeric state of ^{99}Tc at 0.142 MeV primarily (99% probability) decays to another isomeric state at 0.140 MeV. It has a very short half-life (10^{-9} seconds) and therefore decays almost instantaneously to the ground state by the emission of a 0.140-MeV γ-ray or a corresponding conversion electron. The ground state or the nuclide ^{99}Tc itself is a radionuclide. However, its half-life is so long that for all practical purposes it may be considered stable.

other excited state (isomer) of ^{99}Tc, which has an energy of 0.922 MeV, by emission of a β^- particle with E_β max $= 0.45$ MeV. For the remaining 1.4% of the time, the decay takes place to other excited states of ^{99}Tc. The excited state of ^{99}Tc at 0.922 MeV is short lived and quickly ($<10^{-9}$ seconds) decays to the ground state or to lower energy excited states by emission of γ-rays or conversion electrons.

Table 2.1 lists the number of radiations eventually emitted in the decay of ^{99}Mo (β-rays, γ-rays, characteristic x-rays, conversion electrons, and Auger electrons) with their respective energies, $\overline{E}_i$, and the frequency of emission n_i (n_i is defined as the probability of emission of radiation i with energy E_i per decay of a radionuclide). The information given in Table 2.1, however, cannot be obtained from Figure 2.4 alone because additional data and complex computations are required. The Society of Nuclear Med-

icine (New York, NY) has published such information for a large number of radionuclides (MIRD: Radionuclide and Decay Schemes; Weber, Eckerman, Dillman, and Ryman, 1989).

Two more examples of decay schemes, ^{99m}Tc and ^{125}I, are also given here. Appendix A gives in tabular form radiations emitted by a number of other radionuclides commonly used in nuclear medicine. Only those radiations emitted more than 1.0% of the time in the decay are included in these tabulations, which are primarily derived from the above source. For radionuclides not given here or in Appendix A, the reader should consult the above reference. Although information regarding the decay of ^{99m}Tc can be derived from the decay scheme of ^{99}Mo, the decay scheme of ^{99m}Tc is shown separately in Figure 2.5 because of its great importance in nuclear medicine. Table 2.2 lists the relevant data for ^{99m}Tc.

Table 2.2.   Radiations Emitted in the Decay of ^{99m}Tc

Number	Radiation (i)	Frequency of Emission (n_i)	Mean Energy (MeV) ($\overline{E}_i$)
1	γ 1 (conversion electron)	0.986	0.002
2	γ 2 (photon)	0.883	0.140
3	K conversion electron	0.088	0.119
4	L conversion electron	0.011	0.138
5	M conversion electron	0.004	0.140
6	γ 3 (conversion electron)	0.01	0.122
7	K (α) x-ray	0.064	0.018
8	K (β) x-ray	0.012	0.021
9	KLL Auger electron	0.015	0.015
10	LMM Auger electron	0.106	0.002
11	MXY Auger electron	1.23	0.0004

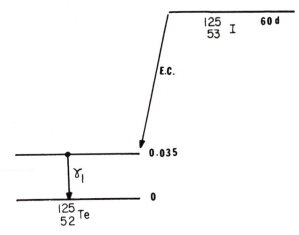

Figure 2.6.   Decay scheme of ^{125}I. ^{125}I decays through electron capture to an isomeric state of ^{125}Te at 0.035 MeV, which subsequently decays to the ground state by the emission of a γ-ray (7% probability) or a conversion electron (93% probability). Because in electron capture and internal conversion a vacancy is created in the K shell, K x-rays of ^{125}Te (29.8 keV) are also emitted in the decay of ^{125}I.

Decay scheme for ^{125}I, a radionuclide widely used in radioimmunoassays, is shown in Figure 2.6. The number of γ-rays, x-rays, conversion electrons, and so on and their respective energies and frequency of emission in the decay of ^{125}I are given in Table 2.3.

It is important to remember that in the decay of ^{99}Mo and ^{125}I, the γ-rays and x-rays emitted are not from ^{99}Mo and ^{125}I nuclides but from ^{99}Tc and ^{125}Te nuclides, respectively, even though in laboratory jargon these are referred to as iodine 125 γ-rays or molybdenum 99 γ-rays. This is a misnomer. The decay actually takes place in the following series:

$$^{99}\text{Mo} \xrightarrow{\beta-} {}^{99}\text{Tc}* \xrightarrow{\gamma} {}^{99}\text{Tc}$$

$$^{125}\text{I} \xrightarrow{\text{K Capture}} {}^{125}\text{Te}* \xrightarrow{\gamma} {}^{125}\text{Te}$$

Table 2.3.   Radiations Emitted in the Decay of ^{125}I

Number	Radiation (i)	Frequency of Emission (n_i)	Mean Energy (MeV) ($\bar{E}_i$)
1	γ 1	0.068	0.035
2	K conversion electron	0.746	0.004
3	L conversion electron	0.107	0.031
4	M conversion electron	0.080	0.035
5	X-ray—K(α)	1.176	0.027
6	X-ray—K(β)	0.240	0.031
7	X-ray—L	0.215	0.004
8	KLL Auger electron	0.137	0.023
9	KLX Auger electron	0.058	0.026
10	KXY Auger electron	0.01	0.030
11	LMM Auger electron	1.49	0.003
12	MXY Auger electron	3.59	0.001

Key Points

1. In a nucleus or a nuclide, the number of neutrons (N) plus the number of protons (Z) equal its mass number (A). A nuclide is represented as $^A_Z X$, where X is the chemical symbol of the element to which this nucleus belongs. Quite often, Z is omitted from the symbol, for example, ^{131}I, which represents a radionuclide of iodine with mass number of 131 (53 protons and 78 neutrons).

2. A nuclide is stable only for certain combinations of Z and N given by the curve of stability (Fig. 2.1). In lighter nuclides, Z = N, and in heavier nuclides, N > Z. Nuclides can also exist temporarily in excited states, called isomers. Whenever an isomer has a half-life of 1 μsec or longer, it is called a metastable state and is denoted with letter m next to the mass number as in ^{99m}Tc.

3. Any other combination of Z and N, away from the stability curve, results in an unstable nuclide (radionuclide).

4. Radionuclides decay through alpha, beta, and gamma processes. In each of these decays, energy, electric charge (Z), and mass number (A) are conserved.

5. In alpha decay, a helium nucleus is given off. The daughter nuclide's mass and atomic numbers are A − 4 and Z − 2, respectively, where A and Z are the parent radionuclide's mass and atomic numbers.

6. In beta decay, an electron or positron is emitted from a nucleus, or an electron is captured from an orbit. In each case, a neutrino is also emitted. Mass number remains unchanged, but atomic number of the daughter nuclide can increase (electron emission) or decrease (positron emission or electron capture) by one unit.

7. In electron capture, a vacancy is created in an orbit. It results in the emission of a characteristic x-ray.

8. In gamma decay, a photon or a conversion electron is emitted. Mass and atomic numbers are not affected. In conversion electron emission, too, a vacancy is formed in the orbit, resulting in emission of characteristic x-ray.

9. Decay schemes summarize the various decay processes and radiations emitted in the decay of a particular radionuclide.

Questions

1. Separate the following nuclides into pairs of isotopes, isobars, isotones, or isomers:

   ^3_1H, ^4_2He, ^3_2He, $^{12}_6C$, $^{12}_7N$, $^{14}_6C$, $^{99}_{43}Tc$, $^{99}_{42}Mo$, $^{99m}_{43}Tc$, $^{100}_{44}Ru$.

2. Identify the following decay processes in which (a) the mass number is unchanged, (b) the atomic number decreases by one, (c) the atomic number increases by one, (d) the mass number decreases by four, and (e) the mass and atomic numbers remain constant.

3. The E_β max for ^3H and ^{32}P are 0.0186 and 1.710 MeV, respectively. What are the average energies of β emission in these decays?

4. In electron capture, an electron is removed from the K or L shell of an atom. Is the daughter atom in the ground state or excited state? Is it ionized?

5. Can a radionuclide decay with all three (alpha, beta, and gamma) processes?

6. What makes two isomers or an isomer and a metastable state different from each other?

7. Find the following radiations in the decay tables given in this chapter or in Appendix A: (a) x-ray with the highest energy in the decay of ^{99m}Tc; (b) γ-rays in the energy range of 100 to 300 keV in the decay of ^{111}In; (c) β-ray with the least frequency of emission, β-ray with the most energy of emission, and γ-rays in the energy range of 700 to 800 keV in the decay of ^{99}Mo; and

(d) % emission and the energies of x-rays in the decay of ^{201}Tl.

In the hypothetical decay scheme shown in Figure 2.7:

8. How many γ_1 and γ_2 will be emitted for 100 disintegrations of radionuclide A and C, respectively? What is the energy of γ_1 and γ_2?

9. Which radionuclide, A or C, can be used as a radionuclidic generator? Identify the metastable state of nuclide B.

10. How many positrons will be emitted in 100 disintegrations of radionuclide C?

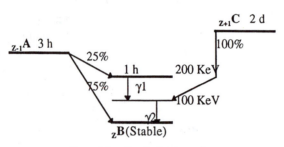

Figure 2.7.   Hypothetical decay scheme.

3 Radioactivity: Law of Decay, Half-Life, and Statistics

Radionuclides are unstable and decay to other nuclides by the processes discussed previously. At what rates do radionuclides decay? Do all radionuclides decay at the same rate? How many radioatoms (i.e., an atom whose nucleus is radioactive) remain after a given period of time? The answers to these and related questions constitute the primary subject matter of this chapter.

RADIOACTIVITY: DEFINITION, UNITS, AND DOSAGE

The number of disintegrations per unit of time (decay rate) is called the radioactivity or simply the activity of a given sample of a radionuclide. For example, if we have a collection of 1000 atoms of a radionuclide at a given time and 50 of these disintegrate in the next 5 seconds, the activity of this sample is $\frac{50}{5} = 10$ disintegrations per second (dis/sec). In algebraic terms, if out of a number N_t of radioatoms at a time t, a number of radioatoms, dN_t, decays in a small time interval dt, the radioactivity, R_t, of the sample is calculated by dividing the number of radioatoms decayed (dN_t) by the interval (dt) during which the decay took place. In other words,

$$R_t = \frac{-dN_t}{dt} \qquad [1]$$

In this equation, the minus sign denotes that the radioatoms are decreasing in number.

The unit of radioactivity is the curie (Ci) in the older system of units (CGS) and the becquerel (Bq) in the newer system of units (SI). SI units are now in the process of replacing the older system of units in scientific work. Unfortunately, in clinical nuclear medicine, old units are still popular. Therefore, I have decided to keep the old units. However, to encourage the use and familiarity of new units, these are given in parentheses for the important data, results, or problems. The major differences between the two systems of units are given in Appendix B.

A curie is defined as the radioactivity of a sample that is disintegrating at a rate of 3.7×10^{10} disintegrations/sec, whereas a becquerel is defined as the radioactivity of a sample that is disintegrating at a rate of 1 disintegration/sec. Because the curie is a large unit, the smaller units derived from it are often used. On the other hand, the becquerel is a small unit, and therefore larger units derived from it are used. Some of these derived units for the curie and the becquerel and their interrelationships are given below:

$$
\begin{aligned}
\text{Curie (Ci)} &= 3.7 \times 10^{10} \text{ dis/sec} \\
&= 37 \text{ GBq} \\
\text{Millicurie (mCi)} &= 10^{-3} \times \text{Ci} \\
&= 3.7 \times 10^{7} \text{ dis/sec} \\
&= 37 \text{ MBq} \\
\text{Microcurie (}\mu\text{Ci)} &= 10^{-6} \times \text{Ci} \\
&= 3.7 \times 10^{4} \text{ dis/sec} \\
&= 37 \text{ KBq} \\
\text{Nanocurie (nCi)} &= 10^{-9} \times \text{Ci} \\
&= 3.7 \times 10 \text{ dis/sec} \\
&= 37 \text{ Bq} \\
\text{Picocurie (pCi)} &= 10^{-12} \times \text{Ci} \\
&= 3.7 \times 10^{-2} \text{ dis/sec.}
\end{aligned}
$$

and

$$
\begin{aligned}
1 \text{Bq} = 1 \text{ dis/sec} &= 27.03 \times 10^{-12} \text{ Ci} \\
&= 27.03 \text{ pCi} \\
\text{Kilobecquerel (KBq)} &= 10^{3} \text{ Bq} = 27.03 \text{ nCi} \\
\text{Megabecquerel (MBq)} &= 10^{6} \text{ Bq} = 27.03 \text{ } \mu\text{Ci} \\
\text{Gigabecquerel (GBq)} &= 10^{9} \text{ Bq} = 27.03 \text{ mCi}
\end{aligned}
$$

In nuclear medicine, the amount of radioactivity (mCi or MBq) administered to a patient is called dosage and not dose (to avoid confusion with another term, radiation dose, discussed in Chapter 7).

LAW OF DECAY

When a sample of a radionuclide is observed for a long period of time, it is found that the radioactivity (R_t) of a sample at a given time (t) depends on the number of the radioatoms (N_t) present at that time and a constant (λ) that is characteristic of a given radionuclide and is different for various radionuclides.

The constant λ, also known as the decay constant, is defined as the probability of decay per unit of time for a single radioatom. Therefore, if there are N_t radioatoms present at time t, then the number of nuclei disintegrating per unit time (R_t) at time (t) will be simply the product of λ and N_t or

$$R_t = \lambda \cdot N_t \qquad [2]$$

From this equation it can be seen that for the different radionuclides (i.e., different λ), the number of radioatoms (N_t) that must be present to produce the same amount of radioactivity (R_t) varies. For example, the number of radioatoms present in a sample of ^{99m}Tc, which has a radioactivity of 1 mCi (37 MBq), is not the same as the number of radioatoms present in a sample of ^{131}I, which has a radioactivity of 1 mCi (37 MBq). This is true because the decay constant for ^{99m}Tc $(\lambda = 3.2 \times 10^{-5}/\text{sec})$ is different from the decay constant for ^{131}I $(\lambda = 10^{-6}/\text{sec})$. The number of radioatoms of ^{99m}Tc or of ^{131}I that must be present in a sample to produce a radioactivity of 1 mCi can easily be determined from equation (2). For ^{99m}Tc,

$$R_t = 1 \text{ mCi (37 MBq)} = 3.7 \times 10^7 \text{ dis/sec and}$$
$$\lambda(^{99m}\text{Tc}) = 3.2 \times 10^{-5}/\text{sec}$$

Therefore, from equation (2),

$$N_t\,(^{99m}\text{Tc}) = \frac{R_t}{\lambda} = \frac{3.7 \times 10^7}{3.2 \times 10^{-5}}$$

$$= 1.15 \times 10^{12} \text{ radioatoms}$$

For ^{131}I,

$$R_t = 1 \text{ mCi (37 MBq) and } \lambda\,(^{131}\text{I}) = 10^{-6}/\text{sec}$$

Therefore, from equation (2),

$$N_t\,(^{131}\text{I}) = \frac{3.7 \times 10^7}{10^{-6}} = 3.7 \times 10^{13}$$

$$= 32 \times N_t\,(^{99m}\text{Tc}) \text{ radioatoms}$$

(i.e., for the same amount of radioactivity, there are approximately 32 times more radioatoms present in a sample of ^{131}I than in a sample of ^{99m}Tc).

Calculation of the Mass of a Radioactive Sample

Once we know the number of radioatoms N_t present in a 1-mCi sample of a radionuclide of mass number A, it is simple to calculate the mass of the radionuclide present in that sample. Here we assume that the radioactive sample contains only the radionuclide under consideration and none of its isotopes.

From equation (2), for a 1-mCi sample, $N_t = \dfrac{3.7 \times 10^7}{\lambda}$. From Avogadro's hypothesis, A grams of this radionuclide contain 6×10^{23} radioatoms. Therefore,

$$\text{the mass of 1 radioatom} = \frac{A}{6 \times 10^{23}} \text{ g}$$

$$\text{or, mass, M, of } N_t \text{ radioatoms} = \frac{N_t \cdot A}{6 \times 10^{23}} \text{ g}$$

or, substituting value of N_t,

$$= \frac{3.7 \times 10^7 \times A}{6 \times 10^{23} \times \lambda} \text{ g/mCi}$$

Mass Number

$$\text{or, mass, M} = 6 \times 10^{-17} \cdot \frac{A}{\lambda} \text{ g/mCi}$$

$$\left[1.67 \times 10^{-8} \frac{A}{\lambda} \text{ g/MBq} \right]$$

EXAMPLE:

What is the mass of a 1-mCi sample of ^{99m}Tc? The mass number for this radionuclide is 99 and the decay constant is 3.2 $\times 10^{-5}/\text{sec}$. Therefore,

$$M = 6.10^{-17} \times \frac{99}{3.2 \times 10^{-5}} = 1.8 \times 10^{-10} \text{ g}$$

Specific Activity

In the above calculations the mass of a 1-mCi sample was determined. In many instances, however, one is interested in the reciprocal of the above (i.e., the amount of radioactivity per unit mass of the radionuclide of interest). This, the radioactivity per unit mass of a radionuclide, is known as the specific activity of a radioactive sample. It is generally expressed in units such as mCi/mg (MBq/mg) or disintegration/min/mg. In the above example, the specific activity of the ^{99m}Tc sample is simply the inverse of M or equal to $1/(1.8 \times 10^{-10})$ mCi/g or equal to 5.5×10^9 mCi/g.

In this example, it was assumed that all atoms of technetium were radioactive and no stable or longer lived technetium atoms were present in the sample. Such a sample that contains only the radionuclide of interest and no other isotope or long-lived radioisotope of that radionuclide is generally called a "carrier-free" sample. Therefore, the above calculation of the specific activity applies only to a carrier-free sample. The specific activity of a sample with carrier (which contains stable or longer lived isotopes of the radionuclide of interest) will always be less than that of a carrier-free sample and will depend on the amount of the carrier in the sample.

When a radionuclide is not present in its elemental form but is a part of a molecule, the concept of specific activity can be generalized to the mass of the molecule rather than the element. For instance, in the above sample, if the technetium radioactivity is present as pertechnetate ($^{99m}TcO_4^-$) rather than as a simple element (^{99m}Tc), one can speak of the specific radioactivity of the sample per unit mass of the pertechnetate. Again, if the sample is carrier free (i.e., no molecules of pertechnetate exist in the sample that does not contain ^{99m}Tc as its part or $^{99}TcO_4^-$ molecules are absent), the specific activity of a pertechnetate sample can be calculated as above by simply taking the inverse of M and substituting the molecular weight of TcO_4^- for A in the above formula. Because the molecular weight of TcO_4^- is about 163, the specific activity of a 1-mCi sample of $^{99m}TcO_4^- = \dfrac{1}{M}$

$$= \dfrac{\lambda}{A \times 6 \times 10^{-17}} = \dfrac{3.2 \times 10^{-5}}{163 \times 6 \times 10^{-17}}$$

$= 3.4 \times 10^9$ mCi/g (1.18×10^{11} MBq/g). Of course, when the sample is not carrier free, the specific activity of the sample will be lower than that of a carrier-free sample and will depend on the amount of carrier present. In nuclear medicine, the knowledge of the specific activity of a sample is important for several reasons. First, the toxicity of a chemical or drug is always dependent on the amount of the chemical or drug administered to the patient. Therefore, it is important to know the amount of a particular chemical or drug in the radioactive sample. Second, the distribution of a radiochemical in a biological system many times depends on the amount of carrier present in the sample. Third, the labeling efficiency of a radionuclide to a chemical is also sometimes dependent on the specific activity of the radionuclide.

The Exponential Law of Decay

If we combine equations (1) and (2), then $-\dfrac{dN_t}{dt} = \lambda\, N_t$. This is a differential equation whose solution is given by the following expression:

$$N_t = N_0 e^{-(\lambda \cdot t)} \qquad [3]$$

This equation relates the number of radioatoms N_t remaining at time t when we initially started (at t = 0) with a number N_0 and is known as the exponential law of decay. If we plot this expression as a linear graph, curves similar to those shown in Figure 3.1 result for different radionuclides (different λ). When one plots the same expression on semilog graph paper, as in Figure 3.2, one obtains straight lines of different slopes (steepness) for different radionuclides.

The exponential law of decay is also true for the radioactivity R_t; that is, R_t is also related to the original radioactivity R_0 by an expression similar to equation (3). This can be seen easily by substituting equation (3) on the right side of equation (2):

$$R_t = \lambda \cdot N_t$$
$$= \lambda \cdot N_0 \cdot e^{-(\lambda \cdot t)} \qquad [4]$$
$$\text{or } R_t = R_0 \cdot e^{-(\lambda \cdot t)}$$

where $R_0 = \lambda \cdot N_0$ is the radioactivity at time 0. If one plots activity R_t as a function of time, curves similar to those shown in Figures 3.1 and 3.2 result.

Half-Life

How does one determine the decay constant λ? Experimentally, it is more convenient to measure another parameter, $T_{\frac{1}{2}}$, known as the half-life. This is defined as the time interval for a given number of nuclei (or their radioactivity) to decay to one-half of the original value. For example, if initially there are 10,000 nuclei in a radionuclide and 5000 of these decay in 5 days, then the half-life of this radionuclide is 5 days. Therefore, by definition of the half-life, when $N_t = \dfrac{N_0}{2}$, then $t = T_{\frac{1}{2}}$.

If we substitute these values in equation (3), we obtain

$$\dfrac{N_0}{2} = N_0 e^{-(\lambda \cdot T_{\frac{1}{2}})}$$

or

$$\tfrac{1}{2} = e^{-(\lambda \cdot T_{\frac{1}{2}})}$$

Because $e^{-0.693}$ is equal to $\frac{1}{2}$ (see Appendix C), it follows that

$$\lambda \cdot T_{\frac{1}{2}} = 0.693 \qquad [5]$$

Equation (5) relates the decay constant to the

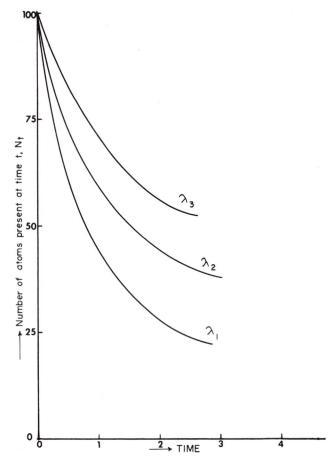

Figure 3.1. Linear plot of the number of radioatoms remaining at a time t as a function of time for three radionuclides with different decay constants: $\lambda_1, \lambda_2, \lambda_3$.

half-life of a radionuclide. From this, if one knows the half-life of the radionuclide, one can calculate the decay constant or vice versa.

EXAMPLE:

Half-life of ^{131}I = 8 days. Determine the decay constant for ^{131}I.

$$T_{\frac{1}{2}} = 8 \text{ days} = 8 \times 24 \times 60 \times 60 \text{ seconds}$$

$$= 0.691 \times 10^6 \text{ seconds}$$

From equation (5),

$$0.691 \times 10^6 \times \lambda = 0.693 \text{ or } \lambda = 10^{-6}/\text{sec}$$

Problems on Radioactive Decay

Equations (1) to (5) are the basic equations necessary for solving routine problems in nuclear medicine. In general, to solve such problems, use of exponential tables is necessary (Appendix C). However, in special cases, where

multiples of half-life are involved, equation (3) can be written in a simpler form by substituting the value of λ from equation (5).

$$N_t = N_0 e^{-\frac{(0.693t)}{T_{\frac{1}{2}}}}$$

$$= N_0 (e^{-0.693})^{\frac{t}{T_{\frac{1}{2}}}} \qquad [6a]$$

$$= N_0 (\tfrac{1}{2})^{\frac{t}{T_{\frac{1}{2}}}}$$

When t is a multiple of $T_{\frac{1}{2}}$, it is easier to make calculations using the above expression than to use exponential tables. For example, if one is interested in finding the number of radioatoms remaining after an interval t = 3 × the half-life of a radionuclide, the above expression becomes

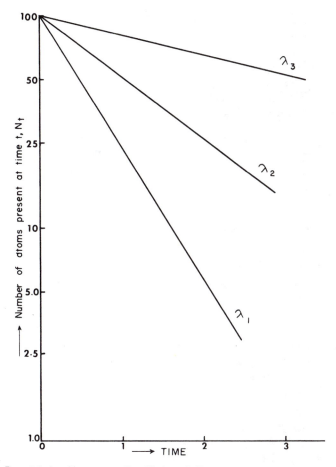

Figure 3.2.   Data as in Figure 3.1 plotted here on a semilogarithmic graph. Plot of exponential function on semilog graph paper results in a straight line. The slope of the straight line is determined by the decay constant or the half-life of the radionuclide.

$$N_t = N_0 \cdot \left(\tfrac{1}{2}\right)^{\frac{3 \times T_{\frac{1}{2}}}{T_{\frac{1}{2}}}} = N_0\left(\tfrac{1}{2}\right)^3$$

$$= N_0/8$$

or one-eighth of the original number. A similar simplification occurs for the activity:

$$R_t = R_0\left(\tfrac{1}{2}\right)^{\frac{t}{T_{\frac{1}{2}}}} \qquad [6b]$$

EXAMPLE 1:
A radioactive sample of ^{99m}Tc contains 10 mCi (370 MBq) radioactivity at 9:00 AM. What will be the radioactivity of this sample at 3:00 PM on the same day? (The half-life of ^{99m}Tc is 6 hours.) In this example,

$R_0 = 10$ mCi (370 MBq)
$T_{\frac{1}{2}} = 6$ hours
$t = 3{:}00$ PM $- 9{:}00$ AM $= 6$ hours

Now, using equation (6b)

$R_t = 10 \cdot \left(\tfrac{1}{2}\right)^{6/6} = 10/2 = 5$ mCi (185 MBq)

EXAMPLE 2:
A preparation of ^{99m}Tc was calibrated at 7 AM and contained 15 mCi/mL (555 MBq/mL) of radioactivity at that time. If the prescribed dosage to the patient is 15 mCi (555 MBq), determine the volume of the preparation that will have to be injected at 10 AM.

$R_0 = 15$ mCi/mL
$T_{\frac{1}{2}} = 6$ hours or $\lambda = \dfrac{0.693}{6}$ /hr
$t = 10$ AM $- 7$ AM $= 3$ hours

Using equations (4) and (5)

$R_t \text{ (at 10 AM)} = 15 \cdot e^{\frac{-0.693 \times 3}{6}} = 15e^{-0.346}$

$= 15 \times 0.70$ (from Appendix C)
$= 10.5$ mCi/mL (388.5 MBq/mL)

Amount desired $= 15$ mCi (555 MBq)

$\therefore \text{Volume needed} = \dfrac{15 \text{ mCi}}{10.5 \text{ mCi/mL}} = 1.43$ mL

EXAMPLE 3:

An iodine-123 capsule is calibrated to contain 100 μCi (3.7 MBq) at noon. However, the capsule is given to a patient early in the morning at 9 AM. Find the dosage of ^{123}I administered to the patient. (Half-life of ^{123}I = 13 hours.)

Let us assume that the radioactivity at 9 AM is R_0. Then, the radioactivity at noon (i.e., 3 hours later) is $R_t = 100$ μCi. Using equations (4) and (5), we get

$$100 = R_0 \cdot e^{\frac{-0.693 \times 3}{13}} = R_0 \cdot e^{-0.16}$$

$$= R_0 \times 0.85 \text{ (from Appendix C)}$$

$$R_0 = \frac{100}{0.85} = 117.6 \text{ μCi (4.3 MBq)}$$

Quite often, the term $e^{-\lambda \cdot t}$ is tabulated for various intervals of time for a given radionuclide. These are known as decay factors. In example 3, the decay factor for ^{123}I for 3-hour decay is 0.85. If the table of decay factors is available, then the relationship of R_t and R_0 becomes simplified as $R_t = R_0 \times$ decay factor, where decay factor $= e^{-\lambda \cdot t}$. Table 3.1 lists some decay factors for ^{99m}Tc.

For practical considerations, a simple fact to remember is that the radioactivity remaining after 10 half-lives of a radionuclide is about one-thousandth of the original radioactivity (i.e., millicurie amounts are reduced to microcurie amounts or MBq amounts are reduced to kBq amounts). This is so because $(\frac{1}{2})^{10} \sim 1/1000$.

Average Life (T_{av})

Occasionally, we encounter the use of another term known as average life of a radionuclide. It is related to the half-life of the radionuclide or the decay constant λ as follows:

$$T_{av} = 1.44 \times T_{\frac{1}{2}} = \frac{1}{\lambda}$$

Because in radioactive decay not all radioatoms decay at the same time, each individual radioatom exists for a different period of time. Average life is therefore the mean of all

Table 3.1.   Decay Factors for ^{99m}Tc

Elapsed Time (hr)	Decay Factor	Elapsed Time (hr)	Decay Factor
0.5	0.94	3.5	0.67
1.0	0.89	4.0	0.63
1.5	0.84	4.5	0.59
2.0	0.79	5.0	0.56
2.5	0.74	5.5	0.53
3.0	0.71	6.0	0.50

these intervals for which individual radioatoms remain in existence.

Biological Half-Life

Under many circumstances, the disappearance with time of a biochemical or drug in a biological system (e.g., thyroid, liver, lungs, bone, blood, plasma, or reticuloendothelial cells) can be described by an exponential law similar to that which holds true for radionuclidic decay. In this case, the disappearance of the biochemical or drug is accomplished through metabolism, excretion, simple diffusion, or some other ill-defined biomechanism. The amount M_t of the biochemical or drug present in the biological system at time t can be determined by an equation similar to that used to determine radioactivity R_t (equation [4]), provided the original amount (M_0) of the biochemical or drug and the probability of its disappearance, λ_{Bio}, in the biological system under consideration is known. In that case,

$$M_t = M_0 e^{-(\lambda_{Bio} \cdot t)} \qquad [7]$$

The disappearance probability, λ_{Bio}, is related to the biological half-life $T_{\frac{1}{2}}(Bio)$, by an equation similar to equation (5):

$$\lambda_{Bio} \cdot T_{\frac{1}{2}}(Bio) = 0.693 \qquad [8a]$$

The biological half-life is defined as the interval during which a given amount of a biochemical or drug in a biological system is reduced to one-half its original value.

Often the disappearance of a biochemical or drug in the biological system cannot be described by equation (7). In these cases, the disappearance of the biochemical or the drug can be described by a sum of several exponential terms as follows:

$$M_t = M_0(A_1 e^{-\lambda^1_{Bio} \cdot t} + A_2 e^{-\lambda^2_{Bio} \cdot t} + \ldots) \qquad [8b]$$

where A_1, A_2 . . . and $\lambda 1_{Bio}$, $\lambda 2_{Bio}$ . . . are constants and are determined experimentally for a given drug in a given biological system.

Effective Half-Life

In nuclear medicine, one is interested in the distribution and the disappearance with time of radioactive substances or drugs from biological systems as a result of both physical decay and biological elimination (metabolism, diffusion, or excretion). Such information is crucial in radiation dose calculations to a patient and to determine the optimum time for imaging after the administration of the radiopharmaceutical.

In the simple case of monoexponential biological distribution and disappearance (equation [7]), the probability of disappearance of a radiopharmaceutical from a biological system is the sum of both the physical and biological disappearance probabilities, i.e.:

$$\lambda + \lambda_{Bio} = \lambda_{eff} \qquad [9]$$

where λ_{eff} is the effective disappearance probability for a radioactive substance or drug. If one converts the various disappearance constants in equation (9) to their respective half-lives, equation (9) becomes

$$\frac{0.693}{T_{\frac{1}{2}}} + \frac{0.693}{T_{\frac{1}{2}}(Bio)} = \frac{0.693}{T_{\frac{1}{2}}(eff)}$$

or

$$\frac{1}{T_{\frac{1}{2}}} + \frac{1}{T_{\frac{1}{2}}(Bio)} = \frac{1}{T_{\frac{1}{2}}(eff)} \qquad [10]$$

From this relationship (equation [10]), one can determine the effective half-life of a radiopharmaceutical if the physical half-life of the radionuclide and the biological half-life of the drug (or chemical) are known. As a rule, however, $T_{\frac{1}{2}}(eff)$ will always be less than or equal to the shorter of the two, $T_{\frac{1}{2}}$ and $T_{\frac{1}{2}}(Bio)$.

In the complex case of biological distribution and disappearance (equation [8a]), it becomes difficult to define a single effective half-life unless each exponential represents a separate biological compartment or organ. Then, each compartment or organ has an effective half-life determined by the physical half-life and the biological half-life for that organ or compartment.

EXAMPLES:

(1) The biological half-life of iodine in human thyroid is about 64 days, and the physical half-life of ^{131}I is 8 days. Determine the effective half-life of ^{131}I in the thyroid.

Given:

$$T_{\frac{1}{2}} = 8 \text{ days}, \quad T_{\frac{1}{2}}(Bio) = 64 \text{ days}$$

Therefore, from equation (10),

$$\frac{1}{T_{\frac{1}{2}}(eff)} = \frac{1}{8} + \frac{1}{64} = \frac{9}{64}$$

or

$$T_{\frac{1}{2}}(eff) = \frac{64}{9} = 7.1 \text{ days}$$

(2) Xenon-133, a radioactive inert gas, is used for lung-function studies. Its physical half-life is 5.3 days and its biological half-life in the lungs is about 0.35 minutes. Determine the effective half-life of ^{133}Xe in the lungs.

Given:

$$T_{\frac{1}{2}} = 5.3 \text{ days} = 5.3 \times 24 \times 60 \text{ minutes}$$
$$= 7632 \text{ minutes}$$
$$T_{\frac{1}{2}}(Bio) = 0.35 \text{ minutes}$$

Therefore, from equation (10),

$$\frac{1}{T_{\frac{1}{2}}(eff)} = \frac{1}{7632} + \frac{1}{0.35}$$

or

$$T_{\frac{1}{2}}(eff) = 0.35 \text{ minutes}$$

In this example, $T_{\frac{1}{2}}(eff) = T_{\frac{1}{2}}(Bio)$. Actually, whenever one of the half-lives, $T_{\frac{1}{2}}$ or $T_{\frac{1}{2}}(Bio)$, is very large (10 times or more) in comparison with the other, then $T_{\frac{1}{2}}(eff)$ is equal to the other half-life ($T_{\frac{1}{2}}(Bio)$ or $T_{\frac{1}{2}}$). In mathematical terms,

$$\text{when } T_{\frac{1}{2}} \gg T_{\frac{1}{2}}(Bio), \text{ then } T_{\frac{1}{2}}(eff) \approx T_{\frac{1}{2}}(Bio)$$

or

$$\text{when } T_{\frac{1}{2}}(Bio) \gg T_{\frac{1}{2}}, \text{ then } T_{\frac{1}{2}}(eff) \approx T_{\frac{1}{2}}$$

STATISTICS OF RADIOACTIVE DECAY

Although λ is defined here as the probability of decay per unit time per atom, in earlier discussions it has been tacitly assumed that the number of radioatoms that decay in time t can be accurately determined. This is not so, nor is there any way to predict exactly which particular atom will decay at a given moment. In practice, the number of radioatoms that decay in a given time t fluctuate around an average value, and for this reason the equations described in the preceding sections express only the relationships of the average values of N_t and R_t.

Because of these statistical variations in nuclear measurements, it is essential to know what contribution these fluctuations make to the total error of a measurement. Barring blunders, error in any measurement has two causes, systematic and random. Systematic errors are caused by the use of miscalibrated instruments and will always either underestimate a measurement or overestimate it depending on which way the error has been made in calibration. Random errors are caused by some uncontrollable factors. Therefore, when a number of repeat measurements are made, these tend to be randomly distributed. The term "accuracy" is used to describe systematic errors, whereas "precision" is used to describe random errors. In radioactivity measurements, random errors that are the result of the natural decay process dominate over the systematic errors and therefore are taken into account only. I should point out here that this discussion of errors is not limited only to counting but is of importance in imaging as well.

Poisson Distribution, Standard Deviation, and Percent Standard Deviation

The probability that a given number of disintegrations (N) will actually occur in a radioactive sample in time t, when the mean number of disintegrations for that sample is N̄, is determined by the Poisson distribution. The mathematical or graphic description of Poisson distribution is complicated. Therefore, it is generally approximated with a Gaussian or standard distribution, shown in Figure 3.3. A Gaussian distribution, which is completely determined by two parameters, mean N̄ and standard deviation σ, is given by the following expression

$$P(N) = \frac{1}{\sigma\sqrt{2\pi}} \cdot e^{-\frac{1}{2}\left(\frac{N-\bar{N}}{\sigma}\right)^2}$$

where P(N) is the probability for observing N disintegrations, N̄ is the average number of disintegrations, and σ is the standard deviation (SD). SD determines the spread or width of a Gaussian (or Poisson) distribution and is commonly used as a measure of random error, or precision, of a radioactive measurement.

A range of $N - \sigma$ to $N + \sigma$ (1 SD) implies that the probability of a given measurement lying within this range is about 68%. When the range is extended to include 2 SDs ($N - 2\sigma$ to $N + 2\sigma$), the probability increases to 95%. Further extension of the range to include 3 SDs ($N - 3\sigma$ or $N + 3\sigma$) increases the probability to 99%.

An important characteristic of Poisson distribution is the relation of its SD to the mean number of disintegrations N̄ as follows:

$$\sigma = \sqrt{\bar{N}} \qquad [11]$$

For large values of N̄, this equation allows a rapid determination of the SD of a given measurement if we replace N̄ by N.

A more useful index of statistical error or precision of a measurement than SD is percent standard deviation (% SD). The % SD of a measurement is determined as follows:

$$\% \, SD = \frac{\sigma}{N} \times 100 = \frac{\sqrt{N}}{N} \times 100 = \frac{100}{\sqrt{N}} \quad [12]$$

This equation states that the precision of a given radioactive measurement can be increased by increasing the observed number of disintegrations. In practical terms, this means that if we measure a radioactive sample for 1 minute and obtain 100 disintegrations during this time, then its % SD, as determined from the above relationship, will be equal to $\frac{100}{\sqrt{100}}$ or 10%. However, if we measure the sample long enough (approximately 100 times longer) so that there are 10,000 disintegrations during this interval, the % SD in this case will be equal to $\frac{100}{\sqrt{10,000}}$ or 1%. In other words, by increasing the time of counting (approximately 100 times), we have decreased the percent error in our results (only by a factor of 10). When the time of counting is

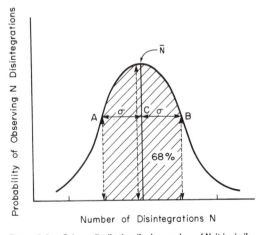

Figure 3.3. Poisson distribution (for large values of N, it is similar to a Gaussian distribution) showing the random nature of radioactivity. The width σ (AC or BC) is known as standard deviation (SD). A range of $N + \sigma$ to $N - \sigma$ (A to B) covers about 68% of the total area of the distribution curve.

limited, a compromise has to be made between the length of counting time and precision.

Propagation of Statistical Errors

In many nuclear applications, we have to add, subtract, multiply, or divide two or more measurements. How does one determine the precision of the final result? To answer this question, let us assume that N1 and N2 are two measurements from which the final result N is obtained by either adding, subtracting, dividing, or multiplying N1 and N2. Without going into detail, then, the % SD of N is given by the following expressions:

When adding: $\% \text{ SD} = \dfrac{100}{\sqrt{N1 + N2}}$ [13]

When subtracting:

$\% \text{ SD} = \dfrac{100 \cdot \sqrt{N1 + N2}}{N1 - N2}$ [14]

When multiplying or dividing:

$\% \text{ SD} = \sqrt{(\% \text{ SD of N1})^2 + (\% \text{ SD of N2})^2}$ [15]

ERROR IN COUNT RATE

Count rate R of a sample is determined by dividing the number of counts N observed in a time interval t by the time interval t or

$$R = \frac{N}{t} \text{ or } N = R \cdot t \qquad (16)$$

Because the error in the measurement of time t is generally very small, the error in R mainly results from the error in N. Therefore,

$$\sigma_R = \frac{\sigma_N}{t} = \frac{\sqrt{N}}{t} \qquad (17)$$

substituting N = R·t from equation (16), we get

$$\sigma_R = \frac{\sqrt{R \cdot t}}{t} = \sqrt{\frac{R}{t}} \qquad (18)$$

To reduce the error of a count rate R, one has to increase the averaging time t. The $\%\sigma_R$ of a count rate is given by the following expression:

$$\%\sigma_R = \frac{\sigma_R \times 100}{R} = \sqrt{\frac{R}{t}} \cdot \frac{100}{R}$$

$$= \frac{100}{\sqrt{R \cdot t}} = \frac{100}{\sqrt{N}} \qquad (19)$$

Room Background

Even when there is no radioactive sample near a radiation detector, it will still record a certain number of disintegrations known as room background. This is due to the presence of minute amounts of radioactivity in the surrounding earth and/or building material. Part of the room background is also contributed by the high-energy radiations of cosmic rays. Room background can be reduced to a low level by shielding the radiation detector. However, it cannot be reduced to zero because of the presence of trace amounts of radioactive substances in the detector and shielding materials themselves and because of the inability to completely shield against high-energy background radiation. In situations where the sample count rate is very low (less than 10 times of background), it is important to take into consideration the room background and its effect on the precision of the final result.

EXAMPLES:

(1) In the thyroid uptake measurement of a patient, it is found that the neck activity gives 900 counts per minute, whereas the standard is 2500 counts per minute. Calculate the % uptake by thyroid and its precision.

$$\% \text{ uptake} = \frac{\text{counts in neck}}{\text{counts in standard}} \times 100$$

$$= \frac{900}{2500} \times 100 = 36\%$$

Using equation (12),

$$\% \text{ SD in neck counts} = \frac{100}{\sqrt{900}} = 3.3\%$$

and

$$\% \text{ SD in standard counts} = \frac{100}{\sqrt{2500}} = 2\%$$

Using equation (15),

$$\% \text{ SD of thyroid uptake} = \sqrt{3.3^2 + 2^2}$$
$$= \sqrt{11 + 4} = 4\%$$

Therefore,

$$\text{Thyroid uptake} = (36 \pm 4\%)\%$$

Because 4% of 36 is 1.4,

$$\text{Thyroid uptake} = (36 \pm 1.4)\%$$

(2) A radioactive sample registers a total (sample + background) of 3200 counts in 1 minute. The room background is 1000 counts per minute. Calculate the net counts of the sample

and the % SD of the total counts, background, and the net counts, respectively.

$$\text{Net counts in the sample} = \text{total counts} - \text{background counts}$$
$$= 3200 - 1000$$
$$= 2200 \text{ counts}$$

Using equation (12),

$$\text{\% SD of the total counts} = \frac{100}{\sqrt{3200}} = 1.7\%$$

and

$$\text{\% SD of the background counts} = \frac{100}{\sqrt{1000}} = 3.1\%$$

Using equation (14),

$$\text{\% SD of the net counts} = \frac{100 \sqrt{3200 + 1000}}{3200 - 1000}$$
$$= \frac{100 \sqrt{4200}}{2200} = 2.9\%$$

This clearly demonstrates the manner in which the room background degrades the precision of a radioactive measurement.

Key Points

1. Radioactivity of a sample is defined as the rate of decay. Its unit is curie (3.7×10^{10} disintegration/sec) in old units and Bq (1 disintegration/sec) in SI units.

2. Radioactivity of a sample at time t, R_t depends on the radioatoms N_t preset at that instant and a characteristic decay constant of the radionuclide, λ and $R_t = \lambda N_t$.

3. N_t and R_t decay with time through law of exponential (i.e., N_t or $R_t = N_0$ or $R_0 e^{-\lambda t}$).

4. Half-life of a radionuclide is related to the decay constant, λ as $\lambda T_{\frac{1}{2}} = 0.693$.

5. Biological half-life and effective half-life are defined in a similar fashion to physical half-life of a radionuclide for a biochemical and a biochemical labeled with a radionuclide, respectively.

6. Radioactive decay is random and follows Poisson statistics. It is impossible to predict how many decays will occur exactly in a given second or minute.

7. Standard deviation (SD) is used to measure the range in which such a decay may lie. This is used to quantify error of a radioactive measurement.

8. For Poisson distribution, SD is related to the average count of a measurement as SD = (average count)$^{\frac{1}{2}}$.

9. One SD range has a 68%, two SD range a 95%, and three SD range a 99% confidence level.

10. When two measurements of radioactivity are added, subtracted, multiplied, or divided, special rules for propagation of errors apply.

Questions

1. Determine the radioactivity of a sample disintegrating at a rate of 10,000 disintegrations per second in (a) millicuries and (b) megabecquerels.

2. What is a 10-mCi dosage of ^{99m}Tc radiopharmaceutical equivalent to in SI units?

3. If the decay constant, λ, of the radionuclide in problem 1 is (a) 0.1 per second and (b) 0.1 per hour, how many radioatoms are present in this sample?

4. Determine the radioactivity of a ^{99m}Tc sample (370 MBq at 0 time) after (a) 9 hours, (b) 12 hours, and (c) 60 hours of decay.

5. How long will it take for the radioactivity of a sample to decay to its 25% value if the radionuclide is (a) ^{201}Tl, (b) ^{99}Mo, or (c) ^{67}Ga?

6. The biological half-life of ^{99m}Tc macroaggregated albumin in the lungs is 6 hours. What is the effective half-life of this agent in the lungs?

7. How many counts are needed to make the standard deviation equal to 1%?

8. A series of 100 1-minute measurements were made, giving an average count rate of 1600 cpm. Of these, how many are in the range of 1600 ± 80?

9. A 99% confidence level of counts taken at the rate of 1200 cpm for 3 minutes is _____ counts.

10. If one obtains 10,000 counts in 5 minutes, what is the standard deviation of the count rate?

4 Production of Radionuclides

In 1896, Henry Becquerel discovered that uranium was radioactive. Soon after, other naturally occurring radionuclides such as radium and polonium were discovered. Most naturally occurring radionuclides have long half-lives (greater than 1000 years) and are not used in nuclear medicine. The radionuclides most commonly used in nuclear medicine (see Appendix D) are artificial, produced by three basic methods:

1. Irradiation of stable nuclides in a reactor (reactor produced);

2. Irradiation of stable nuclides in an accelerator or cyclotron (accelerator or cyclotron produced);

3. Fission of heavier nuclides (fission produced).

METHODS OF RADIONUCLIDE PRODUCTION

Reactor-Produced Radionuclides

A nuclear reactor (for a description of a nuclear reactor, see Fission-Produced Radionuclides, below) is a source of a large number of thermal neutrons. Thermal neutrons are those neutrons whose kinetic energy is very small ($\sim$0.025 eV, which is the kinetic energy of atoms or molecules at room temperature). At these energies, neutrons can be easily captured by stable nuclides because neutrons that are neutral particles do not experience the repulsive coulomb forces of the positively charged nucleus. The capture reaction of neutrons with a given nuclide $^A_Z X$ is represented by either of the following notations:

(i) $^A_Z X + {}^1_0 n \rightarrow {}^{A+1}_{Z} X + \gamma\text{-rays}$
(ii) $^A_Z X (n, \gamma) {}^{A+1}_{Z} X$

In (i), the reactants are to the left of the arrow, and the products of the reaction are to the right. The first equation is written as a chemical reaction; the second equation is a short notation for the same. It can be seen that in the above nuclear reaction, the atomic number (and therefore the chemical nature or element) of the resulting nuclide ($^{A+1}_{Z} X$) does not change; only the mass number, A, increases by 1. Because in this reaction a neutron is being added, the resulting nuclide (if radioactive) quite often decays through β^- emission. I say "if radioactive" because for many neutron capture reactions, the resulting nuclide is stable (e.g., $^{12}_6 C (n, \gamma) {}^{13}_6 C$. In this example, the $^{13}_6 C$ nuclide is a stable nuclide. Another feature of reactor-produced nuclides is that these, in general, are not carrier free. In a carrier-free sample, only the desired radionuclide is present without contamination from its other isotopes. A sample of $^{131}_{53} I$ can be called carrier free only if no other stable isotope or radioisotope of iodine is present in the sample.

Some of the reactor-produced radionuclides, and the nuclear reactions producing them, used in nuclear medicine are given below:

(i) $^{50}_{24} Cr + {}^1_0 n \rightarrow {}^{51}_{24} Cr + \gamma$

^{51}Cr is used for labeling red blood cells and spleen scanning.

(ii) $^{98}_{42} Mo + {}^1_0 n \rightarrow {}^{99}_{42} Mo + \gamma$

^{99}Mo is the source of ^{99m}Tc, which is so commonly used in nuclear medicine.

(iii) $^{132}_{54} Xe + {}^1_0 n \rightarrow {}^{133}_{54} Xe + \gamma$

^{133}Xe is used for lung ventilation studies.

Accelerator- or Cyclotron-Produced Radionuclides

An accelerator or cyclotron is the source of a large number of high-energy (MeV range) charged particles such as p (protons), $^2_1 D$ (deutrons), $^3_2 He$ (helium 3), and $^4_2 He$ (alpha) particles. The classification of an accelerator or a cyclotron depends on the way in which these charged particles are accelerated and is not relevant here. The probability of a nuclear reaction occurring with charged particles is highly dependent on the energy of the bombarding particles. For each charged particle and target, there is a threshold energy below which the nuclear reaction does not occur at all. This is due to the repulsive coulomb forces between the positively charged particle and the positively charged target nuclide. Generally, the threshold energy is in the MeV range. The most common reactions for protons are

(i)
$$_Z^A X + {}_1^1 p \longrightarrow {}_{Z+1}^A Y + n$$

or

$$_Z^A X\,(p, n)\,_{Z+1}^A Y$$

(ii)
$$_Z^A X + {}_1^1 p \longrightarrow {}_{Z+1}^{A-1} Y + 2n$$

or

$$_Z^A X\,(p, 2n)\,_{Z+1}^{A-1} Y$$

The most common reactions for deutrons, $_1^2 D$ (also known as heavy hydrogen), are (in short notations)

(iii) $\quad _Z^A X\,(_1^2 D, n)\,_{Z+1}^{A+1} Y$

(iv) $\quad _Z^A X\,(_1^2 D, p)\,_Z^{A+1} X$

(v) $\quad _Z^A X\,(_1^2 D, 2n)\,_{Z+1}^A Y$

Common nuclear reactions for $_2^3 He$ particles are

(vi) $\quad _Z^A X\,(_2^3 He, n)\,_{Z+2}^{A+2} Y$

(vii) $\quad _Z^A X\,(_2^3 He, p)\,_{Z+1}^{A+2} Y$

Common reactions for α ($_2^4 He$) particles are

(viii) $\quad _Z^A X\,(_2^4 He, n)\,_{Z+2}^{A+3} Y$

(ix) $\quad _Z^A X\,(_2^4 He, 2n)\,_{Z+2}^{A+2} Y$

Most of the above reactions occur in the range of 5 to 30 MeV. As the energy of the bombarding particles further increases, other nuclear reactions occur. Sometimes these additional reactions may also be useful for producing radionuclides. Some radionuclides used routinely in nuclear medicine and produced in an accelerator or cyclotron are given below:

(i)
$$_8^{16} O + {}_2^3 He \longrightarrow {}_9^{18} F + p$$

^{18}F is used for labeling radiopharmaceuticals for positron emission tomography.

(ii)
$$_{30}^{68} Zn + p \longrightarrow {}_{31}^{67} Ga + 2n$$

^{67}Ga is widely used for soft tumor and occult abscess detection.

In the above examples, the radionuclide of interest is formed directly as a result of a particular nuclear reaction. Sometimes, radionuclide of interest may be formed indirectly, by the decay of another radionuclide that is formed first with a nuclear reaction. Two examples of these indirect methods are the production of radionuclides ^{123}I and ^{201}Tl:

(1) Production of ^{123}I

   (i) Nuclear Reaction, $_{52}^{122} Te + {}_2^4 He \longrightarrow {}_{54}^{123} Xe + 3n$ (2 hours, half-life)

   (ii) Decay, $\quad _{54}^{123} Xe \xrightarrow{\text{E.C.}\beta^+} {}_{53}^{123} I$ (13 hours, half-life)

(2) Production of ^{201}Tl

   (i) Nuclear Reaction, $_{81}^{203} Tl + p \longrightarrow {}_{82}^{201} Pb + 3n$ (9.4 hours, half-life)

   (ii) Decay, $\quad _{82}^{201} Pb \xrightarrow{\text{E.C.}} {}_{81}^{201} Tl$ (73 hours, half-life)

Because in charged-particle nuclear reactions the resultant radionuclide generally has an atomic number different from that of the target nuclide, one can chemically separate the two. Therefore, the radionuclides produced by charged particle reactions are generally carrier free. Also, because in these reactions protons are added to a nuclide, these are generally β^+- or K-capturing radionuclides.

Fission-Produced Radionuclides

Soon after the discovery of radioactivity, naturally occurring radioactive nuclides such as $_{88}^{226} Ra$, $_{90}^{232} Th$, or $_{84}^{210} Po$ were found to be good sources of α particles. The reactions of these α particles produced neutrons by $_Z^A X\,(\alpha, n)\,_{Z+2}^{A+3} Y$. When the reactions of the neutrons thus generated were systematically studied, a surprising discovery was made. For many heavier nuclei (A ~ 200), it was found that capture of a neutron, instead of producing a heavier radionuclide, resulted in the production of several radionuclides whose mass numbers were about one-half that of the target nuclide. For example, in the case of ^{235}U, $_{92}^{235} U + {}_0^1 n \longrightarrow {}_{92}^{236} U + \gamma$ seldom occurs. Instead, $_{92}^{235} U + {}_0^1 n \longrightarrow {}_{56}^{141} Ba + {}_{36}^{91} Kr + 4\,{}_0^1 n$ is a much more frequent reaction.

This process of splitting a heavier nucleus into two small nuclei is called fission. Barium and krypton are not the only elements formed in fission. Actually, every element from zinc (Z = 30) to dysprosium (Z = 66) has been identified in fission reaction. Besides the production of radionuclides of intermediate elements (Z = 30 to 66) during fission, another important result is the production of a large number of neutrons (in the above example, 4). A neutron initiates the fission by being captured, yet more than one neutron is produced during fission. These extra neutrons can then cause further fission, thereby producing an even larger number of neutrons. This process is a chain reaction and will theoretically continue until the supply of fissionable material is exhausted. An uncontrolled chain reaction of fissionable material is called an atomic bomb. A controlled chain reaction, however, that is a very good source of a large number of neutrons and of energy (for producing electricity) is known as a nuclear reactor. ^{131}I, so commonly used in nuclear medicine, is produced by fission. Another example of a fission-produced radionuclide is ^{99}Mo, the parent radionuclide of ^{99m}Tc. Like cyclotron- or accelerator-produced radionuclides, fission-produced radionuclides are also generally carrier free.

GENERAL CONSIDERATIONS IN THE PRODUCTION OF RADIONUCLIDES

The amount of radioactivity R_t produced in time t in a nuclear reaction depends on the following factors:

1. The number of bombarding particles/sec/cm^2 known as Flux, I;

2. The total number of the target nuclei irradiated, n × V, when n is the number of the target nuclides in 1 cm^3 and V is the volume of the target material being irradiated;

3. The time of irradiation, t;

4. The half-life or the decay constant of the radionuclide produced (i.e., $T_{\frac{1}{2}}$ or λ);

5. The probability of the given nuclear reaction, called the cross section σ. The unit for cross section is a barn, which is equal to 10^{-24} cm^2.

In the case of neutron capture reactions (reactor-produced radionuclides), the formula relating the above factors to the activity produced after time t is

$$R_t = \sigma \cdot I \cdot n \cdot V \cdot (1 - e^{-\lambda t}) \qquad [1]$$

Because of the factor $(1 - e^{-\lambda t})$, it does not pay to irradiate a target for more than one half-life of the desired radionuclide. In cases where the half-life of the desired radionuclide is sufficiently long (in days), the above equation can be reduced to a simpler form:

$$R_t = \sigma \cdot I \cdot n \cdot V \cdot \lambda \cdot t \qquad [2]$$

A similar equation can be written for charged-particle nuclear reactions. In practice, however, the flux of charged particles is measured as μamp (a unit of electric current) instead of the number per sec/cm^2. In this case, too, the amount of activity produced will depend on the five factors given above. In general, the values quoted for the activity produced by charged-particle reactions are in units of mCi/μamp/hr and are known as the yield of a particular reaction. The higher the yield for a particular nuclear reaction, the easier it is to produce large quantities of the given radionuclide. In selecting the best method of radionuclide production, one has to take into account yield, which is an economical consideration, and purity and the specific activity of the radionuclide, which are biological or scientific considerations and therefore depend on the particular use of the radionuclide.

PRODUCTION OF SHORT-LIVED RADIONUCLIDES, USING A GENERATOR

Because of the reduction in radiation dose to the patient, short-lived radionuclides are often the agents of choice in nuclear medicine. In general, however, the use of short-lived radionuclides entails many problems due to their fast decay. For example, the short half-life of a radionuclide limits the available time for such purposes as processing, transportation, storage, and quality control. For this reason, ^{18}F, with a half-life of 100 minutes, does not have widespread use as a bone-scanning agent. Similar limitations apply to the widespread use of other short-lived radionuclides such as ^{11}C (20.3 minutes), ^{13}N (10 minutes), and ^{15}O (2 minutes), which are quite attractive from other considerations. A radionuclide generator described below (also referred to as a "cow") solves some of the above problems and allows the use of short-lived radionuclides at long distances from the site of production (e.g., a cyclotron or reactor).

Principles of a Generator

A radionuclidic generator is a two- or three-step radioactive series in which a long-lived radionuclide (also called "parent") decays into a short-lived radionuclide (also known as "daughter") of interest.

The following are some examples of radionuclide generators. The first generator system is the most common in use today. The second generator system is useful for geographically remote places where frequent deliveries of the radionuclides are a problem. The third generator is under development and is receiving attention because of its special advantages for positron tomography. The fourth generator produces ^{81m}Kr, which is used in lung ventilation studies sometimes.

(i) ^{99}Mo $\longrightarrow ^{99m}$Tc $\longrightarrow ^{99}$Tc $\longrightarrow ^{99}$Ru

Half-life: 67 hours 6 hours long stable

(ii) ^{113}Sn $\longrightarrow ^{113m}$In $\longrightarrow ^{113}$In

Half-life: 115 days 1.67 hours stable

(iii) ^{68}Ge $\longrightarrow ^{68}$Ga $\longrightarrow ^{68}$Zn

Half-life: 275 days 1.1 hours stable

(iv) ^{81}Rb $\longrightarrow ^{81m}$Kr $\longrightarrow ^{81}$Kr

Half-life: 4.7 hours 13 seconds stable

Figure 4.1. Growth and decay of ^{99m}Tc radioactivity in the decay of ^{99}Mo. It takes about 24 hours for equilibrium to establish. For the solid curve, it is assumed that all disintegrations of ^{99}Mo produce metastable technetium, ^{99m}Tc. The broken curve represents the actual radioactivity of ^{99m}Tc, since only 92% disintegrations of ^{99}Mo produce ^{99m}Tc. The remaining 8% of ^{99}Mo disintegrations produce the ground state, ^{99}Tc, via short-lived isomers.

In a radioactive series, the daughter radionuclide is being continuously produced by the decay of the parent radionuclide and is being continuously destroyed by its own decay. If the half-life of the parent radionuclide is longer than the half-life of the daughter radionuclide, an important phenomenon occurs that is the basis of the generators presently used in nuclear medicine. Under this condition (i.e., $T_{\frac{1}{2}}$ parent $> T_{\frac{1}{2}}$ daughter) and in due course, an equilibrium is established between the parent and daughter radionuclides. In the state of equilibrium, the ratio of the amounts (number of radionuclei present) of the two radionuclides becomes constant. The two radioactivities also maintain a constant ratio (this ratio is in general very close to unity) with time even though the half-lives of the two radionuclides are quite different. In effect, the daughter radioactivity decays with an apparent half-life of the parent radionuclide rather than its own. For example, in a ^{99}Mo-^{99m}Tc generator, the ^{99m}Tc radioactivity in equilibrium with ^{99}Mo decays with a half-life of 67 rather than 6 hours. The growth and decay of the daughter activity in a generator can be exactly predicted using the decay laws given in Chapter 3. Rather than going through complicated mathematics, we showed this relationship graphically in Figures 4.1 and

4.2 for the two most common generators. In both cases, it can be seen that it takes about 4 daughter half-lives to reach equilibrium. For a ^{99}Mo-^{99m}Tc generator, it is about 24 hours, whereas for a ^{113}Sn-^{113m}In generator it is about 6.5 hours. It is also evident from Figures 4.1 and 4.2 that the growth of the daughter radioactivity is not linear with time. Instead, it takes about 1 daughter half-life to reach 50%, 2 daughter half-lives to reach 75%, and 3 daughter half-lives to reach 87% of the equilibrium level.

Once equilibrium has been achieved between the parent and daughter radioactivities, it can be disturbed only by chemical separation (i.e., "milking") of the two radionuclides. After chemical separation, the daughter radioactivity again grows and reestablishes an equilibrium (in about 4 daughter half-lives) with the parent radioactivity, although at a new level. In other words, one has a fresh supply of the daughter radionuclide available for milking each 4 daughter half-lives after the previous milking. However, one does not necessarily have to wait 4 daughter half-lives before milking. Four daughter half-life intervals provide the maximum obtainable yield from a generator. If an emergency supply of the daughter radionuclide is needed, the generator can be remilked sooner. For example, after

Figure 4.2.   Growth and decay of ^{113m}In radioactivity in the decay of ^{113}Sn. It takes approximately 6.5 hours for equilibrium to be established.

1 daughter half-life, remilking will provide about 50% of the maximum obtainable radioactivity of the daughter radionuclide.

The state of equilibrium between the parent and daughter radionuclides is sometimes classified in two categories, transient and secular. When the half-life of a parent radionuclide is not long in comparison with the half-life of the daughter radionuclide, the equilibrium is called transient. ^{99}Mo-^{99m}Tc and ^{87}Y-^{87m}Sr generators are two examples of transient equilibrium. On the other hand, when the half-life of the parent radionuclide is much longer than that of the daughter radionuclide, the equilibrium is termed secular. Two examples of secular equilibrium are ^{113}Sn-^{113m}In and ^{226}Ra-^{222}Rn generators. In secular equilibrium, the activities of the parent and daughter radionuclides become nearly equal, whereas in transient equilibrium, the daughter radioactivity is slightly higher than the parent radioactivity. This distinction between secular and transient equilibrium is of academic interest only, as it carries no practical significance.

Because in the case of a generator a daughter radionuclide is chemically separated from the parent, the daughter radionuclide is produced almost carrier free. I say almost carrier free because the daughter radionuclide, being a metastable state, decays to the same element (e.g., ^{99m}Tc→^{99}Tc). As a consequence and particularly when the generator has not been milked for some time, sufficient amounts of the stable (or almost stable in the case of ^{99}Tc, a long-lived radionuclide) isotope build up in the generator. At the time of milking, this stable isotope will also be milked with the desired radioisotope (e.g., ^{99m}Tc eluate always contains small, but variable, amounts of ^{99}Tc), and therefore such a sample cannot be strictly classified as carrier free.

Description of a Typical Generator

A typical generator is comprised of a glass column filled with a suitable exchange material such as alumina (Al_2O_3). The bottom of the glass column is fitted with a porous glass disk to retain the alumina in the column (Fig. 4.3). The parent radionuclide in equilibrium with its daughter is firmly absorbed on the top of the alumina. The daughter radionuclide is separated (eluted or milked) from its parent ra-

Figure 4.3. Outline of a typical radionuclide generator.

dionuclide by passing a special liquid (eluting solution) through the column at a suitable flow rate. The daughter is dissolved in the eluting solution, whereas the parent is retained by the column.

In a typical ^{99}Mo-^{99m}Tc generator, the column is filled with alumina, ^{99}Mo is part of the molecule, sodium molybdate, and the eluting solution is oxident-free physiologic saline (0.9% sodium chloride solution). The technetium radioactivity elutes in the form of sodium pertechnetate (Na^{99m}TcO$_4$). Molybdenum-99 used in these generators is produced either by irradiation of ^{98}Mo with neutrons or by fission of ^{235}U in a reactor. Molybdenum-99 produced in fission reactions is essentially carrier free and therefore has very high specific activity. On the other hand, ^{99}Mo produced by neutron irradiation of ^{98}Mo is generally of low specific activity. The other difference between these two types of ^{99}Mo is the presence of very minute amounts of other radionuclides (radionuclidic impurities). In the ^{99}Mo produced by neutron irradiation, the most common radionuclidic impurities are ^{134}Cs, ^{60}Co, ^{86}Rb, ^{124}Sb, and ^{95}Zr, whereas in the fission produced ^{99}Mo, the most common radionuclidic impurities are ^{131}I, ^{132}I, ^{89}Sr, ^{90}Sr,

and ^{103}Ru. Because some radionuclides may be eluted with ^{99m}Tc during the milking of the generator, their amounts in the ^{99}Mo sample should be as small as possible.

For any generator system to be of practical use in nuclear medicine, the milking process should be convenient and rapid. The eluate, as described in the next chapter, must be sterile, apyrogenic, and its pH in physiologic range (4.5 to 7.5). In the selection of a suitable generator, one has to consider several other factors such as efficiency, amount of parent breakthrough, radiation shielding, and specific concentration. These factors are discussed below with special reference to the ^{99}Mo-^{99m}Tc generator system.

EFFICIENCY

The efficiency of a generator is defined in the following manner:

$$\text{Efficiency} = \frac{\text{Amount of activity eluted}}{\text{Total daughter activity on the column}} \times 100$$

This is also referred to as the yield of the generator. Present day ^{99}Mo-^{99m}Tc generators give a high yield of ^{99m}Tc, generally between 70 and 90%.

PARENT BREAKTHROUGH

This is the amount of the parent radioactivity that is eluted with the daughter radioactivity. The amount should be as small as possible because any contamination by a long-lived radionuclide (in this case, the parent) increases the radiation dose without providing any benefit to the patient. The maximum allowable level of breakthrough depends primarily on the radiation dose delivered by this contaminant. For the ^{99}Mo-^{99m}Tc generator, the maximum allowable level is 0.15 μCi (5.6 KBq) of ^{99}Mo for each mCi (37MBq) of ^{99m}Tc. In general, the ^{99}Mo breakthrough in ^{99}Mo-^{99m}Tc generators is about $\frac{1}{10}$ of the maximum allowable level. Breakthrough of ^{99}Mo is easily measured with a dose calibrator described in Chapter 8.

CHEMICAL PURITY

Because these generators contain large amounts of alumina, occasionally some aluminum may also be eluted with technetium pertechnetate. Aluminum, depending on its amount, may form colloid. This is an undesirable chemical impurity whose amount should be tested. Its amount should not exceed 10 μg/mL of the eluate. Commercial kits are available to measure simply and quickly the content of aluminum in the eluate.

RADIATION SHIELDING

Because the generators presently in use routinely contain curie amounts of radionuclides, the generator should be properly shielded for the safety of nuclear-medicine personnel. The exact amount of shielding depends on the total amount of radioactivity present and the energy of the γ-rays of the parent and daughter radionuclides. Commercial generators conform to the radiation safety rules and regulations described in Chapter 16.

SPECIFIC CONCENTRATION

This is defined as the number of millicuries per milliliter of the milked eluting solution. This number should be generally high for two reasons:

1. In dynamic studies, such as cardiac or brain blood flow, it is important to have a small concentrated bolus;

2. When labeling a variety of pharmaceuticals with the daughter radionuclide, various dilution steps are required. Therefore, to obtain a reasonably high specific concentration of the labeled compound, it is necessary to begin with a very high specific concentration of the radionuclide. Too high a specific concentration of the radioactivity is, however, of no practical value.

Present generators yield up to 100 mCi/mL specific concentration for ^{99m}Tc.

Key Points

1. Radionuclides used in nuclear medicine are artificial and are produced in a reactor, particle accelerator, or cyclotron.

2. Reactor is a source of neutrons. Most radionuclides produced in a reactor decay through electron emission and contain large amounts of carrier (stable isotope).

3. In some nuclides, capture of neutron leads to fission. In fission, large numbers of carrier-free radionuclides are generated.

4. Particle accelerators or cyclotrons are sources of high-energy charged particles. Radionuclides produced through charged particle reactions decay mainly through positron emission and/or electron capture and are carrier free.

5. Radioactivity produced depends on the amount of target, number of bombarding particles, reaction cross section, time of irradiation, and half-life of the radionuclide being produced.

6. Radionuclidic generators are a source of short-lived radionuclides for hospitals that are some distance away from a reactor or cyclotron. In a generator (^{99}Mo-^{99m}Tc), a long-lived radionuclide (^{99}Mo) decays into a short-lived radionuclide (^{99m}Tc). Under these

conditions, an equilibrium is established in the radioactivities of the parent and daughter radionuclides after a certain interval.

7. The daughter radionuclide can be easily separated from the parent radionuclide. Af-

ter the chemical separation, a new equilibrium is established.

8. Parent breakthrough should be minimum and there are regulatory limits on it. For ^{99}Mo, it is 0.15 μCi/mCi of ^{99m}Tc.

Questions

1. Why do reactor-produced radionuclides generally decay with β^- and accelerator-produced radionuclides with β^+ and/or electron capture?

2. List the factors that determine the amount of radionuclide produced in a reactor or accelerator.

3. Why are carrier-free radionuclides desirable in nuclear medicine?

4. Why is the ^{99}Mo-^{99m}Tc radionuclidic generator so popular in nuclear medicine?

5. Can ^{99m}Tc produced from a generator be strictly considered carrier free?

6. Why is the parent breakthrough in a generator undesirable and to be kept to a minimum?

7. What is the permissible amount of parent breakthrough in the ^{99}Mo$\rightarrow$^{99m}Tc generator?

8. A radionuclidic generator consisting of ^{132}Te (half-life = 78 hours) and ^{132}I (half-life = 3.2 hours) is in transient equilibrium. If the radioactivity of ^{132}Te at this time is 16 GBq, how much radioactivity of ^{132}I will be available 156 hours later if no milking took place during this interval?

9. The above generator is completely milked at 156 hours. The ^{132}I-radioactivity thus obtained is left to decay for 16 hours. How much radioactivity of ^{132}I remained at this time?

10. How often can the above generator be milked for optimum daughter radioactivity?

5 Radiopharmaceuticals

In nuclear medicine, radionuclides are rarely used in their simplest chemical form. Instead, they are incorporated in a variety of chemical compounds that may be of interest because of their favorable biochemical, physiologic, or metabolic properties. A chemical compound tagged with a radionuclide and prepared in a form suitable for human use is known as a radiopharmaceutical. As with all pharmaceuticals, the U.S. Food and Drug Administration (FDA) also approves radiopharmaceuticals for human use.

A radiopharmaceutical is used (with a few exceptions discussed at the end of this chapter) to obtain diagnostic information rather than to produce therapeutic results. It is usually administered in tracer quantities in a single dose and produces no pharmacologic effects.

DESIGN CONSIDERATIONS FOR A RADIOPHARMACEUTICAL

Because a radiopharmaceutical consists of a radionuclide and a biochemical, two considerations apply in designing or developing a radiopharmaceutical, one relating to the radionuclide and the other relating to the biochemical.

Selection of a Radionuclide

To choice of a radionuclide for imaging purposes is chiefly dictated by the necessity of minimizing the radiation dose to the patient and the detection characteristics of present-day nuclear medicine instrumentation.

To minimize the radiation dose to the patient, a radionuclide should have as short a half-life as is compatible with the biological phenomena under study. For example, a radionuclide with a 1 hour half-life, despite its smaller radiation dose, cannot be used in studies of physiologic or metabolic functions that span months. A suggested rule of thumb in this connection is that the physical half-life of the radionuclide should be about $0.693 \times T_{obs}$, where T_{obs} is the time interval between the time of administration of the radionuclide and the time at which measurement

or imaging is to be performed. It should not emit any corpuscular radiations (e.g., β particles, conversion electrons), as these result in a radiation dose to a patient without providing any benefit.

A radionuclide should preferably emit a monochromatic (single-energy) γ-ray with energy between 100 and 300 keV. The upper limit of the desired energy of the γ-ray is the consequence of the detection characteristics of the scintillation camera routinely used to image diagnostic radiopharmaceuticals. As the energy of γ-rays increases, they become more and more penetrating; therefore, a smaller number of them interact within the detector. This reduces the sensitivity of the system. The concept of sensitivity and its importance in nuclear medicine is discussed in later chapters. The lower limit of the desired energy of the γ-ray is arrived at from the consideration of attenuation of γ-rays in the patient. Because γ-rays should be able to penetrate the patient's body effectively, their energy has to be high enough to be transmitted out of the patient's body; hence, the lower limit.

In addition, a radionuclide should be available easily, economically and in an uncontaminated form. Technetium 99m, with its 6-hour half-life and 140-keV γ-ray emission, little emission of corpuscular radiation, and easy economical availability from a generator, comes very close to fulfilling the above requirements. This accounts for its wide use in nuclear medicine.

Selection of a Chemical

Besides being nontoxic in the desired amounts, the choice of the biochemical or pharmaceutical substance in a radiopharmaceutical is dictated by the requirement that it be distributed or localized in the desired organ or compartment and that the uptake by that organ (or part of the organ) in a normal condition differs substantially from uptake in a pathologic condition. This is generally expressed as target to nontarget ratio. The higher the ratio, the higher the contrast in the image and easier it becomes to visualize a disease (see Chapter 13).

To help in the selection of a suitable biochemical, a wealth of information has been acquired in the field of pharmacology. A number of physio-chemical variants determine or affect the distribution and localization of drugs in tissues. Three important determinants in this regard are route of administration, blood flow to the organ or tissues, and extraction by the tissues. Radiopharmaceuticals, with few exceptions, are nearly always administered intravenously, primarily because this is the fastest way to introduce a drug into the circulatory system of the body. Blood flow or perfusion (which can be severely affected in diseases) essentially determines the fraction of the administered dose that will be delivered to a particular organ or tissue during the first transit (10 to 20 seconds). Because blood serves as a carrier for the drug, another property, binding to plasma proteins, plays an important role in the localization of a drug or a chemical in a given tissue. In general, drugs or chemicals strongly bound to plasma proteins remain in blood for a longer period of time (hours to days) and localize to a lesser extent in tissues than those not so tightly bound to plasma proteins.

Extraction of a drug or chemical from circulation and localization in tissue may occur in a number of ways. Simple diffusion, filtration through small pores in the membranes, active transport, receptor binding, and phagocytosis are some examples. It is evident from Table 5.1 that all of these

Table 5.1. Mechanism of Localization of Radiopharmaceuticals

Mechanism	Example
Active transport	Thyroid uptake and scanning with iodine
Compartmental localization	Blood pool scanning with human serum albumin, plasma, or red blood cell volume determinations
Simple exchange or diffusion	Bone scanning with ^{99m}Tc-labeled phosphate compound
Phagocytosis	Liver, spleen, and bone marrow scanning with radiocolloids
Capillary blockade	Lung scanning with macroaggregate (size 8 to 75 μm organ perfusion studies with intra-arterial injection of macroaggregates.
Cell sequestration	Spleen scanning with damaged red blood cells
Receptor binding/ antibody-antigen	Tumor imaging with somatosin receptor-binding ^{111}In-pentetreotide, ^{111}In-OncoScint for tumors

mechanisms were used in the development of the radiopharmaceuticals.

DEVELOPMENT OF A RADIOPHARMACEUTICAL

When appropriate radionuclides and chemicals have been selected, the following steps are involved in the eventual development of a radiopharmaceutical.

Chemical Studies

These are aimed at establishing the best method of radiolabeling the chemical, defining the optimum condition of labeling and in vitro stability, and determining the nature and the extent of the radiochemical impurities.

Animal Distribution and Toxicity Studies

The main purpose of these studies is to determine biodistribution of labeled material and establish safe amounts (radioactivity mainly as the mass of the chemical used is in trace amounts) of the radiochemicals that can be administered to humans without subjecting them to undue risk. Biodistribution establishes the pattern of distribution (major organ or tissues of uptake) of the radioactivity at different times after the administration of the radiochemical in animals considered normal (control) and those in which the appropriate pathologic condition has been induced. From these, one estimates the optimum time for imaging after administration of the radiopharmaceutical and radiation dose delivered to various tissues.

Human or Clinical Studies

Because biodistribution of a radiopharmaceutical in animals may be different from that in humans, initial studies (phase I) in only a small number of humans are performed to establish the distribution patterns, clearance time, mode of excretion, and optimum imaging time for the radiopharmaceutical. In phase II, these studies are extended to include patients with known diseases and provide further evidence of safety and initial proof of the diagnostic or therapeutic efficacy and final estimates of radiation doses to various human tissues. Finally (phase III), a large series of patients are studied that establishes the overall usefulness (i.e., safety and efficacy) of the agent.

Human or clinical studies are performed as an Investigational New Drug under a Notice of Claimed Exemption to the FDA. Once these data are collected, a New Drug Application is submitted to the FDA, which must approve it before its commercial use.

QUALITY CONTROL OF A RADIOPHARMACEUTICAL

Because all radiopharmaceuticals are intended eventually for human use, strict quality control is very important. To ensure optimum quality, the following properties of a radiopharmaceutical must be considered.

Radionuclidic Purity

Ideally, the radiopharmaceutical should contain only the desired radionuclide. Often, however, it is not possible to avoid some contamination by other radionuclides, and therefore it is essential to hold this contamination to a low level. A contaminating radionuclide does not add to diagnostic information, but it does increase the radiation dose to the patient and, in many cases, may degrade the image quality. A good example is provided by the radionuclide, ^{123}I, which is difficult to produce without ^{124}I as radiocontaminant. Iodine-124, besides significantly increasing the radiation dose to the patient, degrades image quality because of its emission of high-energy γ-rays.

The amount of impurity is generally given as μCi (KBq) of radiocontaminant per μCi (KBq) or mCi (MBq) of the desired radionuclide. Sometimes the limit of the allowable contamination is set by governmental agencies, as in the case of ^{99m}Tc, for which the amount of ^{99}Mo must not exceed more than 0.15 μCi for each mCi of ^{99m}Tc. In cases where no such limits are prescribed, the rule of thumb is to keep the radiation dose to the patient from the radiocontaminants to less than 10% of that due to the radionuclide of interest.

Another important aspect of radionuclidic purity is that it does not stay constant with time. Where the half-life of the desired radionuclide is shorter than that of the radiocontaminant, radionuclidic purity degrades with time and vice versa. For example, because the half-life of ^{124}I, a common radiocontaminant in ^{123}I, is longer than ^{123}I, the radionuclidic purity is best at the time of the production of this radionuclide, and as the radionuclide is stored, it becomes progressively less pure.

The most common method of determining the nature and extent of radionuclidic impurity is with gamma spectroscopy using a NaI (Tl) or Ge (Li) detector, both of which are discussed in Chapter 8.

Radiochemical Purity

Because a radionuclide may form several compounds with a given chemical, it is important to ascertain that a given radiopharmaceutical is in the desired chemical form. Any radiochemical impurities present should be precisely stated. In this regard, it is also important to consider that although a radiochemical may be pure to begin with, it may not be stable over a period of time as a result of the action of radiation or the nature of the chemical itself. To avoid this deterioration, the radiochemical should be stored properly according to the instructions of the manufacturer. For example, radioiodinated human serum albumin (RIHSA), which, among other things, is used as a blood pool scanning agent, may be 99.9% pure when freshly prepared. With time, however, some of the radioiodine becomes free. The amount of free radioiodine strongly depends on storage conditions. The contamination with free radioiodine is several times higher if RIHSA is stored at room temperature than if it is refrigerated. A significant amount of free radioiodine will interfere with the intended study.

A common method for the detection of radiochemical impurities is thin-layer or paper chromatography.

Chemical Purity

A radiopharmaceutical should contain only the desired chemical. In the final preparation of the radiopharmaceutical, there may be a number of chemicals involved besides the radiochemical of interest. These chemicals should be compatible with each other in vitro and safe for the patient. In addition, these must not distort the in vivo function of the main chemical. Aluminum breakthrough in a ^{99}Mo-^{99m}Tc generator is an example of potential chemical impurity.

Sterility

A radiopharmaceutical should be sterile (i.e., free from any microbial contamination) and therefore should be tested to this effect before use in patients. In the case of radiopharmaceuticals using short-lived radionuclides (^{99m}Tc and ^{113m}In), where prior testing of the final product is not feasible, the sterility of the labeling technique should be tested adequately and periodically.

Apyrogenicity

Even if the preparation is sterile, it may still contain pyrogens that, when intravenously administered to a patient, may cause a reaction. A radiopharmaceutical, therefore, should also be tested for pyrogenicity before use in humans. If this is not feasible, as in the case of short-lived radionuclides, the apyrogenicity of the technique should be ascertained properly and periodically.

LABELING OF RADIOPHARMACEUTICALS WITH TECHNETIUM-99m

Because of the very attractive physical characteristics of ^{99m}Tc, a variety of chemicals have been labeled with this radionuclide despite the fact that the exact mechanism of technetium labeling with these compounds is often not known. Technetium-99m, in the form of sodium pertechnetate ($Na^{99m}TcO_4$), is easily obtained in the laboratory from a ^{99m}Mo-^{99m}Tc generator. The labeling of most chemicals by ^{99m}Tc is achieved by first reducing the pertechnetate to ionic technetium (mostly Tc4+) and then complexing it with the desired chemical. The common agent used for reducing purposes is stannous chloride ($SnCl_2$). Because the half-life of ^{99m}Tc is short (6 hours), most labeling has to be performed "in-house." This is greatly simplified by the use of sterile and pyrogen-free kits, in which all the desired chemicals are premixed and held together in a lyophilized state under an inert atmosphere (nitrogen gas) except the radionuclide (hence, quite often referred as "cold kit"). To label a particular chemical compound, it is necessary only to introduce a known

amount of sterile and pyrogen-free sodium ^{99m}Tc pertechnetate into the kit vial; the labeled compound is ready to use within a few minutes.

Three parameters—labeling efficiency, in vitro stability, and in vivo stability—are important considerations in the selection of a kit. Labeling efficiency is defined as the percent of total radioactivity present in the kit that is tagged to the appropriate molecule or compound. For most kits currently in use in nuclear medicine, labeling efficiencies under optimum conditions are in excess of 90%, sometimes even reaching as high as 99%. The remainder of the radioactivity (which is not tagged to the desired compound) is present as radiochemical impurity. In kits that use $SnCl_2$ as the reducing agent, radiochemical impurities are, in general, of two forms, free pertechnetate (which was not reduced) and reduced or hydrolyzed technetium (which was reduced but did not tag to the compound of interest). Reduced or hydrolyzed technetium sometimes forms a colloid with excess tin present in the kit. This is also a radiochemical impurity but in a different form.

The in vitro stability of a labeled compound determines the time it can be stored on the shelf without significant deterioration. A high in vitro stability allows the compound to be labeled once and then used in a number of patients at different times of the day. Both labeling efficiency and in vitro stability of compounds prepared from kits can be maximized by observing a few simple precautions such as using only oxident-free sodium pertechnetate solution and ensuring no air (oxygen in air, being an oxidizer, reacts with the reducing agent and thus competes with pertechnetate for the reducing agent) is introduced into the reaction vial during the labeling procedure. The in vitro stability of a kit can also be extended by the use of preservatives in the reaction vial as is done by some manufacturers and/or by storing the labeled material at low temperatures. I should caution here that in vitro stability of a labeled compound is different from in vitro stability of the cold kit or the chemical compound itself.

The in vivo stability of a labeled compound determines how closely the distribution of the radiolabeled compound in the biological system parallels that of the unlabeled compound. The distribution of a labeled compound should be similar to the unlabeled compound at least for the duration of the study.

TECHNETIUM-99m-LABELED RADIOPHARMACEUTICALS

The distribution and use of the most common technetium-labeled compounds in nuclear medicine are described below. Most of these compounds can be easily and rapidly prepared from the commercially available kits.

Technetium-99m Pertechnetate ($^{99m}TcO_4^-$)

This radiopharmaceutical is obtained directly from the ^{99}Mo-^{99m}Tc generator using saline as the eluting solution. In biological systems, it behaves similarly to iodine. After oral or intravenous administration, it is selectively concentrated in the thyroid, salivary glands, stomach, and choroid plexus. Disappearance of the pertechnetate from plasma is a multiexponential function. About 50% of the compound is rapidly diluted into extravascular spaces within 15 to 20 minutes. The remaining amount disappears from the plasma with a half-life of about 3 hours. About 20 to 30% of the injected dose is excreted eventually in feces at a slow rate.

Stomach, which is the major organ of uptake, contains 20 to 25% of the injected dosage at 4 hours. So much radioactivity remains in the stomach even after 24 hours that it is not advisable to perform imaging of an abdominal organ using ^{99m}Tc-labeled radiopharmaceuticals (or whose principle gamma emission is 170 keV or below) on a patient who had imaging performed with ^{99m}Tc pertechnetate up to 48 hours before the intended study.

Technetium 99m pertechnetate is presently used for thyroid, salivary gland, and stomach imaging. It is no longer used as a brain imaging agent.

Technetium-99m-Labeled Sulfur Colloid

This radiopharmaceutical is easily prepared using commercially available kits. Colloids in general are removed from the bloodstream by the reticuloendothelial (RE) cells of the body. The relative distribution of the colloids among the RE cells of the various organs depends on factors such as the size, nature, and amount of colloidal particles; blood supply to the organ; and on other physiologic and pathophysiologic considerations. In the case of colloidal sulfur tagged with technetium-99m (particle size ~0.3 μm), about 70 to 80% of the injected dosage is localized in the liver within 10 to 20 minutes of intravenous administration. Of the remaining amount, about 3% is deposited in the spleen and about 15 to 20% is localized in the bone marrow. This agent is, therefore, primarily used for liver, spleen, and bone marrow imaging.

Another ^{99m}Tc-labeled compound sometimes used for liver, spleen, and bone marrow imaging is albumin microaggregates (particle size ~1 μm).

Technetium-99m-Labeled Macroaggregated Albumin (^{99m}Tc MAA)

This radiopharmaceutical is primarily used in lung imaging. Within a few seconds after intravenous administration of ^{99m}Tc MAA, 90 to 95% of the injected dosage is trapped in the capillary and precapillary bed of the lungs. For effective lung localization, the albumin macroaggregates must be between 15 and 75 μm in size. The biological half-life of ^{99m}Tc MAA in the lungs is about 8 to 12 hours. The ^{99m}Tc albumin macroaggregates are broken down in smaller (micro) particles that are then taken up by the RE cells of liver and spleen.

Technetium-99m-Labeled Polyphosphate, Pyrophosphate, and Diphosphonate

These radiopharmaceuticals are primarily used for bone imaging. After an intravenous injection, about 50 to 60% of the injected dosage is localized in the skeleton within 15 to 20 minutes. The remainder of the dose is distributed in soft tissue and plasma from which it is excreted slowly in the urine. About 20 to 30% of the injected dose is either excreted or taken up by the kidneys within 3 hours of the injection. Of these three groups, polyphosphate has the slowest plasma clearance and is therefore the least desirable for bone imaging. Methylene disphosphonate has the fastest plasma clearance of these compounds.

Use of ^{99m}Tc pyrophosphate and ^{99m}Tc diphosphonate for the detection of myocardial infarctions is now well established.

Technetium-99m-Labeled Human Serum Albumin

This radiopharmaceutical is primarily used for blood pool imaging such as heart or placenta. After intravenous administration, it is retained in the plasma for a long period of time. However, ^{99m}Tc-labeled albumin is not as stable in vivo as albumin labeled with radioiodine or radiochromium. Therefore, it is not the preferred agent for plasma volume determination.

Technetium-99m-Labeled Red Cells

Labeling of red cells with radionuclides, in general, is a complex and time-consuming procedure. Recently, however, a simple and expeditious method has been developed to label red cells in vivo with ^{99m}Tc. This has increased the popularity of ^{99m}Tc-labeled red cells over that of ^{99m}Tc-labeled albumin for blood pool scanning, particularly for heart. In this method, two steps are involved. In step 1, a patient's red cells are coated with stannous ion (Sn^{2+}). This is achieved simply by injecting about one-fifth of a "cold" pyrophosphate kit into the patient. A cold kit is a preparation reconstituted using saline only (i.e., without any radioactivity). In step 2, performed about 30 minutes later, the desired amount of the ^{99m}Tc radioactivity in the form of pertechnetate is administered to the patient as a second injection. The "pretinned" red cells in the patient quickly reduce the pertechnetate to ionic technetium that then readily binds to the red cell surface. Little free pertechnetate or reduced technetium remains in circulation. Most radioactivity (90%) is bound to the patient's red cells.

The second step—tagging of ^{99m}Tc to the pretinned red cells—can also be performed in vitro by withdrawing pretinned red cells from the patient and incubating them with the desired amount of ^{99m}TcO$_4^-$. The red cells thus labeled may be heat damaged, if desired, by heating them in a water bath at 50°C for half an hour. Damaged red cells are used to image the spleen, without interference from the liver, which is the case when sulfur or other colloids are used to image the spleen.

Technetium-99m-Labeled 2,3-Dimercaptosuccinic Acid (DMSA)

This radiopharmaceutical is the agent of choice when morphology of the renal cortex is of interest. After an intravenous administration, this radiopharmaceutical is quickly mixed with the plasma volume from where it is cleared with a half time of about 1 hour. By 2 hours, between 40 and 50% of the injected dosage is taken up by the renal cortex and about 15% is excreted in urine. Because of rapid in vitro decomposition of ^{99m}Tc-labeled DMSA, it should be stored in a refrigerator and used within half an hour of labeling.

Technetium-99m-Labeled Diethylenetriamine Pentaacetic Acid (DTPA)

This radiopharmaceutical is used primarily for kidney imaging. After intravenous administration, ^{99m}Tc DTPA is rapidly cleared by the kidneys. The biological half-life in plasma of DTPA chelates in humans is about 15 minutes. Over 80% of the injected dosage can be recovered in urine between 2 and 3 hours postinjection.

Technetium-99m-Labeled Glucoheptonate

Biological behavior of this radiopharmaceutical is somewhere between that of (^{99m}Tc) DTPA and (^{99m}Tc) DMSA. Its clearance from plasma is slower than that of ^{99m}Tc DTPA but faster than ^{99m}Tc DMSA. Maximum uptake by renal cortex, which is reached at about 1 hour postinjection, is about 25% of the injected dose. Another 25% of the injected dosage is excreted in urine by this time. This radiopharmaceutical is primarily used for renal imaging. Another use of this radiopharmaceutical is in detection of myocardial infarctions at an early stage (within 2 to 3 days postinfarction). At this early stage, ^{99m}Tc pyrophosphate is not useful for the detection of myocardial infarctions.

Technetium-99m-Labeled Mertiatide (MAG3)

This compound has recently been introduced to study renal function and serves as a substitute for iodohippuran. After intravenous injection, this compound is rapidly cleared by the kidneys through both active tubular secretion and glomerular filtration. In normal subjects, 90% of the injected dosage can be recovered in urine. This compound, even though bound to plasma proteins, has a fast plasma clearance because of the reversible nature of the binding.

Technetium-99m-Labeled 2,6-Dimethyl Acetanilide Iminodiacetic Acid (HIDA) and Related Compounds (Diethyl-IDA, PIPIDA, and DISIDA)

These radiopharmaceuticals are used for imaging the hepatobiliary system. In normal subjects, ^{99m}Tc HIDA is rapidly cleared from blood by hepatocytes. The half time for blood clearance is approximately several minutes. The transit of the radioactivity from the liver through gallbladder to the intestine is also fast. Within an hour after administration, over 70% of the injected dosage is in intestine. About 15% of the injected dosage is excreted in urine during the first hour. The remainder of the activity is eventually excreted in feces. Urinary excretion of diethyl-IDA is smaller than that of PIPIDA or DISIDA. The transit and excretion of these compounds through the hepatobiliary system is strongly dependent on the patency of this system.

Technetium-99m-Labeled Sestamibi (Cardiolite)

This compound is primarily used in the imaging of the heart. Its use in tumor imaging (e.g., in breast) is also being explored. Being a technetium-labeled compound, it has an advantage over thallium for heart imaging in terms of providing higher photon flux for the same radiation dose to the patient. After intravenous injection, it is extracted by the myocardium in proportion to the blood flow. Its first-pass extraction efficiency is slightly less than that for thallous ion, but it does not redistribute and remains in the myocardium up to 3 hours post injection, thus providing a long time for planar imaging and single-photon emission computed tomography (SPECT). The liver and kidneys are other organs of large localization (20 and 14%, respectively).

It is excreted intact through the hepatobiliary system and the kidneys.

Technetium-99m-Labeled Teboroxime (Cardiotec)

This is another technetium-labeled compound for imaging the myocardium. After an intravenous injection, it is rapidly cleared from the blood. The peak activity in the myocardium is achieved within a few minutes, after which it starts to redistribute. This fact is its strength and its weakness—strength because it allows rest and stress studies to be performed in less than an hour, a marked improvement over Sestamibi, and weakness because there is not enough time to get good quality planar images and almost no time to perform SPECT. The liver is the organ with maximum localization, 33% at 15 minutes postinjection. The primary route of excretion is the hepatobiliary system, with some excretion through the kidneys.

Technetium-99m-Labeled Tetrofosmin (Myoview)

This is the most recent radiopharmaceutical approved for heart imaging. After an intravenous injection, it is rapidly cleared by skeletal muscle, heart (1%), liver (7.5%), and kidneys (6.2%). Less than 5% of the injected dosage remains in blood. Salivary and thyroid glands also show elevated concentrations. Within 48 hours of administration, 75% of the dose is excreted from the body (40% urine and 35% fecal excretion). Excretion, particularly from the skeletal muscle, is increased significantly during exercise. This agent allows the exercise and rest heart scans to be performed on the same day (exercise scan followed 4 hours later with rest heart scan).

Technetium-99m-Labeled Brain Imaging Agents (Exametazime [Ceretec], Hexamethylpropylene-amine Oxime [HMPAO], and Ethyl Cysteinate Dimer [ECD])

These radiopharmaceuticals cross the blood-brain barrier and therefore actively localize in the brain. Because their uptake is generally a function of regional blood flow, these agents, in conjunction with SPECT, are now being used to measure brain function. After an intravenous injection of Ceretec, the peak uptake (7%) in the brain is reached at 1 minute. The remainder of the dosage is distributed in the whole body, particularly in muscle and soft tissues. It is excreted from the body by way of the gastrointestinal tract and the kidneys in similar amounts.

RADIOIODINE-LABELED RADIOPHARMACEUTICALS (^{131}I AND ^{123}I)

With the advent of technetium-99m-labeled compounds, use of iodine-131-labeled compounds for imaging has declined sharply. However, two radioisotopes of iodine, ^{123}I and ^{131}I, are commonly used for diagnosis of thyroid disease. ^{131}I is also used in the treatment of hyperthyroidism and thyroid cancer. For diagnostic purposes, ^{123}I (13-hour half-life and 87% 160-keV γ-ray emission) is the radionuclide of choice because it delivers significantly less radiation dose to the thyroid than ^{131}I. The two disadvantages of ^{123}I are its cost and, sometimes, the presence of large amounts of other radioisotopes of iodine such as ^{124}I. These contaminants not only increase radiation dose but also degrade image quality.

Iodine-131- or Iodine-123-Labeled Sodium Iodide

The radiopharmaceutical, ^{131}I- and ^{123}I-labeled, sodium iodide is commercially available as a capsule or solution with high specific activity and is almost carrier free. Because iodine ion is readily absorbed from the stomach, it is generally administered orally. After an intravenous administration, the iodide ion is very quickly distributed throughout the extracellular water. From there, it is slowly taken up by the thyroid, stomach and intestine, salivary glands, and choroid plexus. A large fraction is filtered into the urine by the kidneys. By 24 hours, about 75% of the injected dose is excreted, 15% taken up by thyroid, 4 to 5% is in the gastrointestinal tract, and 1 to 2% is circulating in the blood. In the thyroid, iodine is then organified and produces thyroid hormones such as T_3 or T_4. The distribution of radioiodide can be drastically changed in some disease states, particularly hyperthyroidism or severe kidney malfunctions. In hyperthyroidism, thyroid can take up to 90% of the administered dosage with practically no excretion, whereas in hypothyroidism, thyroid takes up little (sometimes less than 1 to 2%) iodide with excretion increased up to 95%.

Other Iodine-123-Labeled Radiopharmaceuticals

Two other ^{123}I-labeled compounds, ^{123}I-Hippuran and ^{123}I-isopropylamphetamine (Spectamine), are finding increased use in nuclear medicine. Iodine-123-Hippuran is rapidly cleared by the kidneys and therefore is used to study renal function in the form of renograms that can be obtained either using dual scintillation detector probes or by imaging with a scintillation camera interfaced with a computer. Iodine-123-isopropylamphetamine is used for measuring brain function, particularly the changes in regional brain-blood flow. Brain function studies with ^{123}I Spectamine in conjunction with SPECT are promising as an alternative to the use of ^{18}F deoxy-glucose in conjunction with positron emission tomography, which necessitates an in-house cyclotron and associated paraphernalia.

COMPOUNDS LABELED WITH OTHER RADIONUCLIDES

Gallium-67 Citrate

This radiopharmaceutical is used in detection of soft tissue tumors and inflammatory diseases. After an intravenous administration, a significant fraction of the gallium in blood (30%) is bound to plasma proteins—in particular, to transferrin. The remainder of the gallium quickly diffuses into extracellular spaces and is slowly cleared by the kidneys. By 24 hours, about 15% of the dosage is excreted in urine and about 10% is circulating in the blood. The remainder of the radioactivity is distributed in kidneys, bone, liver, and lymph nodes. Biological half-life of gallium in humans is between 1 and 2 weeks. Therefore, significant amounts of this radionuclide persist in body even after 2 weeks. Besides excretion in urine (about 25% in 1 week), there is significant (10%) excretion in stool that sometimes interferes in interpretation of images of the abdominal area. The exact mechanism of localization of ^{67}Ga in tumors or inflammatory lesions is not well established at this time.

Thallous-201 Chloride

This radiopharmaceutical is primarily used for detection of myocardial infarction and/or ischemia. Thallous ion mimics the biological behavior of potassium, which is avidly localized intracellularly. Like potassium, immediately after intravenous injection thallous ion quickly leaves the circulation ($T_{\frac{1}{2}}$ = 4 minutes) and is taken up by various organs generally in proportion to the blood supply of the given organ (brain is one exception where there is almost no accumulation). At about 15 to 20 minutes, 4% of the injected dosage is localized in myocardium, 12% in liver, 4% in kidneys, and the bulk of the remainder is distributed in muscles throughout the body. Biological half-life of thallous ions in humans is about 10 days. Its use for myocardial imaging is based on the fact that its cellular uptake is dependent on blood flow to that region and the integrity of the cells themselves. Therefore, reduced uptake of thallous ion in a region is either a reflection of reduced blood flow (ischemia) or a reflection of damage to the cells (infarction).

Chromium-51-Labeled Red Cells

These are used to determine the red cell volume and red cell mean life. Because labeling of red cells has to be performed in-house for each patient, this is a complex procedure. First, blood is withdrawn from the patient. It is then incubated with acid dextrose (ACD) and sodium chromate-51 solution at 37 to 39°C for 10 minutes. Chromate ion readily penetrates the red cell membrane. Inside the cell it is reduced to Cr^{3+}, which has high affinity for hemoglobin. Small amounts of chromate ion that do not enter the red cells are then reduced to Cr^{3+} outside the cells by addition of appropriate amounts of ascorbic acid. The blood-ACD-ascorbic acid solution is now ready to be injected back into the patient. Only the labeled red cells remain in circulation. Small amounts of $^{51}Cr^{3+}$ not bound to the cells are quickly excreted in urine by the kidneys.

Indium-111-Labeled DTPA

This radiopharmaceutical is presently the agent of choice for imaging cerebrospinal fluid dynamics. When injected intrathecally, it rises to the basal cisterns within 2 to 3 hours. By 24 to 48 hours, radioactivity rises over the convexities of the brain and into the parasagittal area. There, it is resorbed into blood and quickly excreted by the kidneys into urine.

Indium-111-Labeled Platelets and Leukocytes

These are used for thrombus and abscess detection, respectively. The technique of platelet or leukocyte labeling with radionuclides is quite involved because it first requires separation of platelets or leukocytes from other components of blood. Once platelets or leukocytes have been separated, they can be labeled with ^{111}In by incubating them with ^{111}In oxine at room temperature for 30 minutes. Because of the involved preparation of ^{111}In-labeled platelets or leukocytes, these have not found widespread use in nuclear medicine.

Indium-111-Labeled-DTPA Pentetreotide (OctreoScan)

This radiopharmaceutical has been recently introduced in clinical nuclear medicine for the detection of somatosin receptor-containing tumors. After an intravenous injection, this is rapidly cleared from blood (30% of the injected dosage in blood at 10 minutes postinjection). It is distributed throughout the soft tissues but has higher concentrations in kidneys, spleen, and liver (7, 2.5, and 2% at 4 hours, respectively). Pituitary and thyroid glands also exhibit high concentrations. It is mainly eliminated from the body through urinary excretion (85% in 24 hours). Imaging is performed at 24 hours postinjection.

Radiolabeled Monoclonal Antibodies

Wide interest exists in the possible use of monoclonal antibodies and their fragments, labeled with different radionuclides, for diagnosis and therapy of cancer and its metastases. Because of the affinity of tumor antibodies for tumor antigens, a high degree of localization occurs in tumors when antibodies labeled with radionuclides are injected into patients. This localization can be used for diagnosis by labeling antibodies with radionuclides such as ^{111}In and ^{99m}Tc or for therapy with [131]I. Because antibodies are basically proteins, their blood clearance is generally slow and is similar to radiolabeled human serum albumin. Two antibodies, one labeled with [111]In (OncoScint) and the other labeled with [99m]Tc (CEA-Scan), were recently approved by FDA for clinical use. Several more (^{111}In-labeled ProtoScint and ^{99m}Tc-labeled Verluma) are on the way.

RADIOACTIVE GASES AND AEROSOLS

Of all the radioactive gases used in nuclear medicine, ^{133}Xe has found the most popularity because of its easy availability and useful physiologic properties. It can be used in a gaseous form or as a saline solution. In a gaseous form, it is used for lung ventilation studies; in a saline solution administered intravenously, it is used for lung perfusion studies. When ^{133}Xe is injected intra-arterially in a saline solution, it can be used to measure the blood flow to the organ supplied by that artery. Biological half-life of xenon in the body is only a few minutes. Only a very small component (~2%), probably the portion that is transferred to fat in the body, has a much longer biological half-life (~10 hours).

Recently, with the commercial availability of [81]Rb-[81m]Kr generators, many institutions have started using [81m]Kr instead of [133]Xe. Because of the 13-second half-life of [81m]Kr, repeat studies can be performed in the same patient within a few minutes of the first study.

Also, use of ^{99m}Tc DTPA aerosols for such purposes is now well documented. Commercially available nebulizers produce ^{99m}Tc-labeled aerosols with particle sizes ranging from 1 to 3 μm for lung ventilation studies. About 90% of the aerosol remains airborne and the remainder is removed from the lungs rapidly.

THERAPEUTIC USES OF RADIOPHARMACEUTICALS

The main concern of nuclear medicine is diagnostic applications of radionuclides. Here, we briefly discuss some therapeutic uses of radiopharmaceuticals when they are administered internally to a patient.

Design of a Radiopharmaceutical for Therapeutic Uses

Physiologic and biochemical considerations in designing a radiopharmaceutical for therapeutic purposes are similar to those that apply in designing a radiopharmaceutical for diagnostic uses; the primary objective in both cases is a high target to nontarget ratio. For therapeutic uses, a diseased cell is the target.

Because the objective of therapeutic use of a radiopharmaceutical is to kill diseased cells with radiation, the physical requirements for a radionuclide are the opposite of those desired for diagnostic purposes. The radionuclide should emit only particulate radiation (α- or β-ray) and preferably no penetrating radiation (x- or γ-ray).

Problems and Uses

The main problem arising in the treatment of a patient with internally administered radionuclides is the calculation of the radiation dose (rads) to the target. Accurate calculations of the radiation dose require accurate data about the physical decay characteristics of the radionuclide and its distribution in the body (see Chapter 7). Although accurate data are available with regard to the first parameter, accurate data with regard to the latter are difficult to obtain, particularly in the case of a patient who is about to be treated. Usually, a tracer dose is administered to a patient for this purpose. From the blood disappearance, the urinary and fecal excretion rates, and the relative distribution in the body of this tracer dose, as determined by area imaging or SPECT where possible, an estimation is made of the various parameters to be used in the calculation of radiation dose. Unfortunately, even these parameters may not describe the behavior of the therapy dosage (100 to 1000 times larger than the trace dosage); therefore, the resulting radiation dose from a therapy dosage may be quite different from that estimated from the trace or diagnostic dosage. Another unpredictable factor in such treatment is the variability of the biological response of different individuals to the same radiation dose.

Despite this inability to deliver the exact number of rads to a target by internal administration of the radionuclides, success has been achieved for the treatment of a number of diseases. Table 5.2

Table 5.2.   Therapeutic Uses of Radiopharmaceuticals

Radionuclide and Chemical Form	Dosage (mCi) and Route of Administration	Dosage (MBq)	Uses
^{131}I as iodide	3–10 oral	111–370	Hyperthyroidism
^{131}I as iodide	50–200 oral	1850–7400	Cancer of thyroid
^{32}P as orthophosphate	3–20 intravenous	111–740	Polycythemia, bone metastases, and leukemia
^{90}Sr as strontium chloride	3–5 intravenous	111–185	Bone metastases
^{32}P, ^{198}Au, ^{90}Y, ^{177}Lu in colloidal form, particle size ranging from 0.01 to 50 μm	10–150 intravascular, intracavitary, and interstitial	370–5550	A variety of malignant diseases

summarizes the present status of the therapeutic uses of internally administered radionuclides.

MISADMINISTRATION OF RADIOPHARMACEUTICALS

Radiopharmaceuticals, at rare occasions due to human error, can be administered in more amounts, in a different form, or through a different route than prescribed. In either case, the U.S. Nuclear Regulatory Commission (NRC) or comparable state agency, which regulates the use of FDA-approved radiopharmaceuticals and other uses of radionuclides, has defined what constitutes a misadministration. These are divided into three categories: the two radioisotopes, ^{125}I and ^{131}I, *in the form of sodium iodide;* all *other diagnostic radiopharmaceuticals;* and all *other therapeutic radiopharmaceuticals.*

1. ^{125}I *and* ^{131}I, *in the form of sodium iodide:* (a) Administration of a dosage greater than 1.1 MBq (30 μCi), or to a wrong patient, or through a wrong route and/or (b) whenever the administered dosage exceeds the prescribed dosage by more than 20% and the difference is greater than 1.1 MBq (30 μCi).

2. All *other diagnostic radiopharmaceuticals:* (a) Administration of a wrong radiopharmaceutical, or to a wrong patient, or through a wrong route and/or (b) the radiation dose from the administered amount of radioactivity is more than 50 mSv (5 rems) effective dose equivalent or 500 mSv (50 rems) dose equivalent to any individual organ (radiation dose is described in Chapter 7).

3. All *other therapeutic radiopharmaceuticals:* (a) Administration of a wrong radiopharmaceutical, or to a wrong patient, or through a wrong route and/or (b) when the dosage differs from the prescribed dosage by more than 20%.

After the discovery of misadministration, the NRC or appropriate state agency has to be notified no later than the next calendar day. Then a written report has to be submitted within 15 days providing the cause of misadministration and corrective actions taken and proposed.

These regulations are published in Title 10, part 35 of the Code of Federal Regulations (10CFR35) and should be consulted for more details.

Key Points

1. Radiation dose and the available detection instruments determine the characteristics of an ideal radionuclide to be used in nuclear medicine. An ideal radionuclide emits no particle radiation, emits an x- or γ-ray of energy in the range of 100 to 300 keV, and has a short half-life.

2. Pharmaceutical principles determine the localization of radiopharmaceuticals in

tissues. These are active transport, compartmental localization, simple exchange or diffusion, phagocytosis, capillary blockade, cell sequestration, and receptor binding.

3. Radiopharmaceuticals have to satisfy quality control standards for radionuclidic purity, radiochemical purity, chemical purity, sterility, and apyrogenicity.

4. Commercial kits available for labeling with

^{99m}Tc should be tested for two chemical impurities, ^{99m}TcO$_4^-$ and reduced or hydrolyzed ^{99m}Tc.

5. Labeling with ^{99m}Tc dominates the radiopharmaceuticals used in nuclear medicine for diagnostic purposes.

6. The radionuclide, ^{131}I, dominates the therapeutic uses.

QUESTIONS

1. List the ideal properties of a radionuclide to be used for diagnostic purpose.

2. Three radionuclides with the following properties are available to you: (a) $T_{\frac{1}{2}}$ = 3 minutes, γ emission (70%) of 180 keV energy; (b) $T_{\frac{1}{2}}$ = 1 day, γ emission (100%) of 250 keV energy, a small fraction of conversion electrons (5%); (c) $T_{\frac{1}{2}}$ = 2 days, γ emission (20%) of 300 keV, β emission with a maximum energy of 2.0 MeV. Which one of these is best suited for (a) tumor localization when the optimum tumor uptake occurs at 18 hours post injection, (b) blood perfusion in an organ, and (c) radiation therapy?

3. List the factors that affect the localization of a radiopharmaceutical in tissue.

4. Does strong plasma binding of a radiopharmaceutical (a) help, (b) hinder, or (c) have no effect on the rate of uptake by a tissue?

5. What happens to the radionuclidic purity with time if the half-life of the desired ra-

dionuclide is longer than that of the radiocontaminant?

6. What are the two most common radiochemical impurities in a ^{99m}Tc-labeled radiopharmaceutical?

7. How does the presence of oxygen interface with labeling of a pharmaceutical with ^{99m}Tc?

8. List the various radiopharmaceuticals that are used for imaging the following organs: liver, bone, bone marrow, myocardium, blood pool, kidneys, lungs, hepatobiliary system, thyroid, spleen, tumors, and brain.

9. How do the roles of the two agencies, FDA and NRC, differ in regulating the radiopharmaceuticals?

10. What is the maximum time interval between the discovery of misadministration and its written notification to the appropriate agency?

6 Interaction of High-Energy Radiation With Matter

Interaction is a fundamental aspect of nature. Our ability to see, hear, smell, and taste is a vivid manifestation of interaction. This chapter, however, focuses on the mechanism of interaction of high-energy radiation with matter. Radiation in this context is used in a general sense. It encompasses both corpuscular radiation (e.g., charged particles and neutrons) and electromagnetic radiation in the form of x- and γ-rays.

The material presented here is basic to an understanding of the detection and effects (especially biological) of high-energy radiation and of protection against it. Because the subject matter is complex, only the salient features are presented. For ease of presentation and understanding, this chapter has been divided into three sections: (1) interaction of charged particles (with energies of 10 keV to 10 MeV) such as e, e^+, p, α, and ^2D; (2) interaction of high-energy photons such as x- and γ-rays; and (3) interaction of neutrons.

INTERACTION OF CHARGED PARTICLES (10 keV TO 10 MeV)

Principal Mechanism of Interaction

When a charged particle passes through a substance (target) it interacts with the negatively charged electrons and positively charged nuclei of the target atoms or molecules. Through the coulomb forces, it tries to attract or repel the electrons or nuclei near its trajectory. As a result of these pushes and pulls (a sophisticated name for these is inelastic collisions), the charged particle loses some of its energy, which is taken up by the electrons of the target atoms near its trajectory. The absorption of energy by the target atom leads to its ionization or excitation. In this energy range (10 keV to 10 MeV), ionization events predominate over excitation events. For this reason, high-energy radiations are sometimes referred to as ionizing radiations, although excitation events are by no means negligible. The probability of inelastic collisions in general is so high that it does not take a material of much thickness to stop the charged particles completely.

Differences Between Lighter and Heavier Charged Particles

Do all charged particles interact in a similar way? The answer is yes and no. Yes, because inherently the nature of interaction for all charged particles in this energy range is the same (inelastic collisions). No, because the manifestation of these interactions on lighter particles—whose masses are of the order of an electron (e.g., e and e^+)—and heavier particles—whose masses are equal to or more than that of a proton (e.g., p and α)—is strikingly different. Lighter particles in inelastic collisions with the electrons of the target atoms, besides losing energy, tend to be deflected at larger angles than the heavier particles. This leads to a wide variation in the paths of the two kinds of particles (depicted graphically in Figure 6.1 for an electron and proton). The path of a heavier particle is more or less a straight line, whereas that of a lighter particle is more tortuous (zigzag). Whenever a lighter charged particle is deflected at a large angle, the energy transferred to the target electron is also quite large. As a result, the target electron acquiring this large amount of energy also behaves like a high-energy charged particle, thus creating its own path in the target medium. The paths created by high-energy secondary electrons are known as δ-rays. These are shown by the dotted lines in Figure 6.1. In the case of a proton or other heavier particles, this type of energy transfer is rare.

Range, R, of a Charged Particle

As a charged particle travels farther and farther in a medium, it loses more and more energy and therefore more and more of the target atoms close to its path become ionized or excited. Eventually, the charged particle loses all its kinetic energy and comes almost to a halt. The average distance traveled by a charged particle in the incident direction is defined as its range, R. This definition of range, R, is strictly valid only for heavy charged particles such as α particles. For lighter particles, it is difficult to define the range, R, exactly. For our purpose, it is sufficient to think of the range, R, of

Figure 6.1.   Range, R, of a charged particle. Heavy charged particles (e.g., protons) travel and lose their energy in more or less straight lines. Light charged particles (e.g., electrons) lose their energy in a zigzag fashion. Lighter charged particles can transfer large amounts of energy in a single encounter with an electron of the medium, thus creating what are known as δ-rays. Plus and minus signs represent the ionization of the atoms of the medium. (Figure not to the scale as electrons will travel much farther than protons.)

light particles such as electrons or positrons as the minimum thickness of a material that they are just unable to penetrate. The concept of the range of a charged particle is quite useful in radiation protection, design of radiation detectors, and radiation dosimetry.

The range, R, of the heavier charged particles, because they travel more or less in straight lines, is nearly equal to the average path length of the charged particles in a given medium, whereas the range, R, for the lighter particles such as electrons, because of their more tortuous paths, is much shorter than the average path length (Figure 6.1). Table 6.1 lists the ranges of α particles and electrons for various energies and mediums, providing a rough idea of the distances involved.

The concept of range is sometimes used with

β-emitting radionuclides in which β particles are emitted with varying amounts of energy up to a maximum, E_β max. In this case, the range is more or less determined by E_β max.

Factors That Affect Range, R

The range, R, of a charged particle depends on various factors. Four of the most important of these are described below.

ENERGY (E)

The range, R, of a given particle increases with increase in the initial energy, E, of the particle. For example, the range of a 5-MeV electron is about six times longer than that of a 1-MeV electron. The exact relationship of R to E is complex, but in the energy range of our interest, R is linearly related to the initial energy of the charged particle E or R = AE + B, where A and B are constants.

MASS (M)

Lighter particles have longer ranges than heavier particles of the same energy and charge. The range of a 1-MeV positron (e^+) is much longer than the range of a 1-MeV proton (p^+, 2000 times the mass of an e^+). Mass dependence of the range is sometimes expressed as velocity dependence. A 1-MeV positron is traveling at a much higher speed than a 1-MeV proton. The range, R, of a charged particle increases as the velocity of the charged particle increases.

CHARGE (Q)

A particle with less charge travels farther than a particle with more charge. For example, a ^3_1H (charge 1; mass 3) particle has a longer range than a ^3_2He (charge 2; mass 3) particle of the same energy. The exact relationship is R$\alpha \frac{1}{Q^2}$.

Table 6.1.   Approximate Ranges of Charged Particles

	Range, R (cm)			
	Soft Tissue		Air	
Energy (keV)	e or e$^+$	α	e or e$^+$	α
10	2×10^{-4}	$< 10^{-5}$	1.6×10^{-1}	1×10^{-2}
100	2×10^{-2}	1.4×10^{-4}	16	1×10^{-1}
1,000	4×10^{-1}	7.2×10^{-4}	3.3×10^2	5×10^{-1}
10,000	5	1.4×10^{-2}	4.1×10^3	10.5

Therefore, $^3_1$H particle travels four times the distance of $^3_2$He particles. The signs of the charge (positive or negative) do not affect the range.

DENSITY OF THE MEDIUM (D)

The range, R, of a charged particle strongly depends on the density of the medium through which it is traversing. The higher the density of the medium, the shorter the range of a charged particle, that is, R is inversely proportional to the density, d, of the medium or R$\alpha \frac{1}{d}$. For this reason, the ranges of charged particles are always much longer in gases than in liquids or solids.

Bremsstrahlung Production

Besides losing energy through inelastic collisions, charged particles can lose energy through the "bremsstrahlung" process. In this case, when a charged particle in the electric field of a nucleus experiences a sudden acceleration or deacceleration, it sometimes emits high-energy photons (x-rays). The probability of such interaction in the energy range of our interest is indeed very small except when electrons and positrons interact with high atomic-number materials (e.g., lead, steel). The fraction of energy, f, released as x-rays by electrons of energy E (MeV) in a material with atomic number Z is given approximately by the following equation:

$$f = \frac{Z \cdot E}{1400} \quad \text{(E is in MeV)}$$

In an x-ray tube with a tungsten target (Z = 74) and electrons with 100-keV incident energy, only 0.5% of the total energy of the electrons is converted into x-rays. The same fraction (0.5%) of the total energy of the electrons is converted into x-rays when a 1-MeV electron passes through water (Z = 7.4) except that the x-ray spectrum (energies of emitted x-rays) in this case is quite different from that produced in the first case (x-ray tube). For the purposes of nuclear medicine, because production of high-energy photons by this mechanism is generally very small, it is therefore ignored.

Stopping Power, S

Quite often, instead of using the range, R, of a charged particle, another parameter known as stopping power, S, is used. Stopping power is defined as the ratio of the amount of energy lost (dE) by a charged particle in traversing a small distance (dx) in a given medium to the distance dx, or

$$S_{medium} = -\frac{dE}{dx}$$

The range, R, is related to the stopping power in an approximately inverse relationship (i.e., the higher the stopping power of a given medium, the shorter will be the range of a given particle in that medium). Because of this relationship, the stopping power, S, also depends on the same factors (E, M, Q, and d) on which the range, R, depends, although now the relationships are approximately inverse to that of the range, R.

Linear Energy Transfer

Linear energy transfer (LET) is an important parameter in radiation biology. It is defined as the ratio of the amount of energy transferred (dE_{local}) by a charged particle to the target atoms in the immediate vicinity of its path in traversing a small distance (dx) to the distance dx, or

$$LET = -\frac{dE_{local}}{dx}$$

Difference Between LET and Stopping Power, S

In discussing stopping power, S, one is concerned with the total energy lost by the particle, whereas in discussing LET one is concerned with the local (immediate vicinity of the track) deposition of energy by the charged particle. Because of this, S and LET are almost equal for heavier particles. For lighter particles, however, the two quantities differ significantly because of the energy lost in the δ-rays or through the bremsstrahlung process, which does not deposit energy locally. Both the stopping power, S, and LET are measured in the same units (keV/μm).

Annihilation of Positrons

There is no difference in the way in which an electron or a positron loses energy in a medium. However, a positron, once it has lost its energy, is not stable and is quickly annihilated by combining with an electron. The mass energy of the electron and the positron is converted into two γ-rays of 511 keV that travel in opposite directions. Remember that the annihilation of positron occurs only when it has lost almost all of its energy (i.e., near the end of its range in a medium).

INTERACTION OF X- OR γ-RAYS (10 keV TO 10 MeV)

Although a photon does not have any electrical charge, it nevertheless interacts with electrical charges and therefore with matter that is composed of electric charges. The probability of interaction and the modes of interaction of a photon with matter are strongly dependent on the energy of the photon. Here we are interested only in the interaction of high-energy photons (x- or γ-rays) with matter.

The probability of interaction of an x-ray or γ-ray with an atom is, in general, very small compared with that of high-energy charged particles. As a consequence, x- or γ-rays have more penetrating power than high-energy charged particles. Because of this high penetrating power of x- or γ-rays, it is not practical to use concepts such as stopping power or range. Instead, new concepts known as linear attenuation coefficient (μ[linear]) and the half-value layer (HVL) are commonly used.

Attenuation and Transmission of X- or γ-Rays

Let us consider a simple experiment in which a parallel beam of x- or γ-rays of a given energy (E_γ) is incident on a thin slab of 1-cm^2 cross section and x-cm thickness (Fig. 6.2). When a γ-ray passes through this slab, three things may occur: the γ-ray may be completely absorbed by the material, the γ-ray may be deflected (scattered) with some or no loss of energy, or the γ-ray may pass through the slab without any interaction. The first two processes together are known as attenuation; the third is known as transmission. The transmission of γ-rays of a given energy, E_γ, through a thickness, x, in the above experiment depends only on the nature of the material (density and atomic number) and the thickness, x, of the slab. For a given material, the dependence on the thickness, x, can be experimentally determined by measuring the number of γ-rays (those without any loss of energy or deflection) transmitted through different thicknesses of the slab. The data resulting from

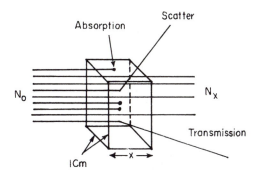

Figure 6.2.   Attenuation of γ-rays. When a flux, N_0, of γ-rays is incident on a substance of x-cm thickness, a smaller flux, N_x, is transmitted by the substance. The remaining γ-rays either are absorbed by the substance or are scattered out from the incident beam.

such an experiment can be accurately related by the following mathematical expression:

$$\frac{N_x}{N_0} = e^{-\mu(\text{linear})x} \qquad [1]$$

where N_0 and N_x are, respectively, the number of γ-rays incident on the slab and transmitted through a thickness, x, of the slab. The linear attenuation coefficient, μ(linear), represents in physical terms the probability of the interaction of a γ-ray passing through a unit area of a material 1-cm thick; μ(linear) strongly depends on the γ-ray energy (E_γ) and the nature of the material (density and atomic number). Note that equation (1) is mathematically the same as that for radioactivity decay with time (see p. 21, Chapter 3). However, here it is describing a completely different physical process—namely, the transmission of γ-rays through a thickness, x, of a given material. The energy dependence of the linear attenuation coefficient of four substances useful for our purpose is shown in Figure 6.3.

Experimentally, it is easier to determine the parameter known as the HVL than to determine μ(linear). HVL is defined as the thickness of a material that attenuates one-half of the incident γ-rays. Referring to equation (1), when

$$\frac{N_x}{N_0} = \frac{1}{2}, \quad x = \text{HVL}$$

HVL is related to μ(linear) by the following expression:

$$\text{HVL} = \frac{0.693}{\mu(\text{linear})} \qquad [2]$$

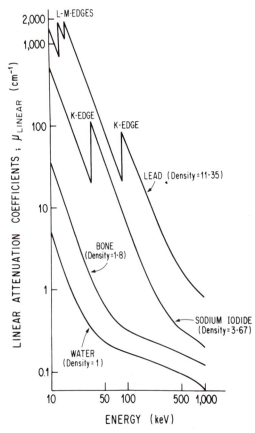

Figure 6.3. Linear attenuation coefficient, μ(linear), of water, bone, sodium iodide, and lead as a function of x- or γ-ray energy.

which is similar to that for the half-life of a radionuclide ($T_{\frac{1}{2}}$) and its decay constant, λ. The parameter μ(linear) is measured in units of cm^{-1}, whereas HVL is expressed in cm. Once HVL or μ(linear) is known, one can easily determine the parallel beam attenuation of γ-rays through any thickness, x, of a material using equation 1 or one of the shortcuts described in Chapter 3 (p. 22) for solving problems involving exponentials.

EXAMPLE:

The half-value layer of a 140-keV γ-ray in a NaI(Tl) crystal is approximately 0.3 cm. Determine the percentage of γ-rays transmitted through a 1.2-cm ($\approx \frac{1}{2}''$) thick NaI(Tl) crystal for a 140-keV γ-ray parallel beam.

A thickness of 1.2 cm is expressed as $\frac{1.2}{0.3} = 4$ HVL of a 140-keV γ-ray in a NaI(Tl) crystal. Because for 1 HVL the ratio of $\frac{N_x}{N_0} = \frac{1}{2}$, for 4 HVL the ratio will be $\frac{N_x}{N_0} = \left(\frac{1}{2}\right)^4$

$= \frac{1}{16}$; therefore, the percentage of γ-rays transmitted is $\frac{100}{16}$

or 6%. In other words, 94% of the γ-rays will be attenuated. Here, the thickness, x, is a multiple of HVL; therefore, it is not necessary to use equation (1).

Mass Attenuation Coefficient, μ(mass)

Because μ(linear) is dependent on the density of the absorbing material, it is often important to know the mass attenuation coefficient, μ(mass), that removes the effect of the density from the linear attenuation coefficient. The mass attenuation coefficient reflects the probability of an interaction with a unit mass of a material. The mass attenuation coefficient is related to the linear attenuation coefficient by the following expression:

$$\mu(\text{mass}) = \frac{\mu(\text{linear})}{\text{density}}$$

The units for μ(mass) are expressed as $\frac{cm^2}{gm}$.

Atomic Attenuation Coefficient, μ(atom)

The two probabilities of interaction, μ(linear) and μ(mass), describe the interaction of γ-rays at the macroscopic level (1 g or 1 cm^3). How does one relate these two quantities to those at the atomic level (e.g., the probability of γ-ray interaction with one atom, μ[atom])? The number of atoms in 1 g of a substance can be determined by dividing Avogadro's number (N_{av}) by the atomic weight (A), that is, number of atoms in 1 g $= \frac{N_{av}}{A}$. Then μ(atom) can be determined by dividing μ(mass) by the number of atoms in 1 g of that substance:

$$\mu(\text{atom}) = \mu(\text{mass}) \bigg/ \frac{N_{av}}{A} = \frac{\mu(\text{mass}) \cdot A}{N_{av}}$$

The units for μ(atom) are expressed as cm^2.

Mechanisms of Interaction

We described the attenuation of x- or γ-rays without, thus far, specifying the mechanisms that cause this attenuation. In this energy range (10 keV to 10 MeV), there are three basic processes through which a photon interacts with matter: photoelectric effect, Compton effect, and pair production. The relative importance of each type of interaction depends on the energy of the photon and the atomic number of the material with which it is interacting.

A salient feature of x- or γ-ray interaction with matter via any of the above three mechanisms is the production of a high-energy charged particle (electron or positron) that then loses energy in the medium by producing ionizations and excitations as previously discussed. Because of this, x- or γ-radiation is sometimes known as indirectly ionizing radiation.

PHOTOELECTRIC EFFECT

When an incident photon interacts with a target atom through the photoelectric effect, it transfers all its energy to one of the electrons in the atom (i.e., the photon is completely absorbed by the atom), as shown in Figure 6.4. The absorption of energy by the atom leads to its ionization by the emission of an electron, which acquires kinetic energy (Ee) in an amount equal to that of the photon energy (Eγ) minus the electron's binding energy in the shell (B.E.; i.e., Ee = Eγ − B.E. of the electron). The electron can be released from any atomic shell. If it is released from one of the inner shells (e.g., K) a vacancy is created in this shell that is subsequently filled by

an electron from one of the higher shells (e.g., L, M), as described in Chapters 1 and 2. This results in the emission of a characteristic x-ray or Auger electron by the atom. If, on the other hand, outer-shell electrons are involved in the photoelectric interaction, the atom is simply ionized. The probability of the photoelectric interaction by an atom, τ(atom), strongly depends on two factors: the energy of the photon Eγ and the atomic number (Z) of the atom involved in the interaction.

Dependence on Eγ

The probability of photoelectric interaction, τ(atom), decreases sharply with the increase in the x- or γ-ray energy. It is inversely proportional to the cube of γ-ray energy, that is, $\tau(\text{atom}) \propto \frac{1}{E_\gamma^3}$. Therefore, the probability of a γ-ray of 45 keV interacting through the photoelectric effect is eight times higher than for a γ-ray of 90-keV energy, that is, $\frac{(90^3)}{(45^3)} = 8$.

There is, however, one exception to this inverse cube law. Whenever the energy of the γ-ray (Eγ) becomes equal to the binding energies of the electrons in the various atomic shells of an atom, the probability of photoelectric interaction rises sharply. For example, the probability of the photoelectric interaction of a 45-keV γ-ray with a lead atom should be eight times higher than that of a 90-keV γ-ray according to the $\frac{1}{E_\gamma^3}$ rule.

However, because the binding energy of the electrons in the K shell of a lead atom is about 88 keV, the probability of a photoelectric interaction of 90-keV γ-ray increases to a point where it almost becomes equal to that for a 45-keV γ-ray. The probability of photoelectric interaction of an 80-keV γ-ray in lead is about six times lower than that of a 90-keV γ-ray despite the fact that the latter is a higher energy γ-ray. The regions where the $\frac{1}{E_\gamma^3}$ law does not hold are called absorption edges, and their occurrence depends on the atomic number, Z, of the atom with which the γ-ray interacts. For example, the K absorption edge (where K-shell electrons are involved) occurs at approximately 88 keV in lead but at only 32 keV in iodine (Fig. 6.3).

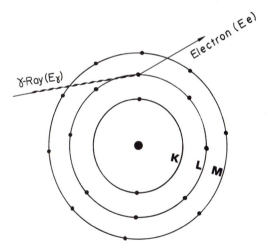

Figure 6.4. Photoelectric interaction. A γ-ray transfers all its energy to an orbital electron of the absorbing material atom and thereby ionizes the atom. The electron thus released carries an amount of energy, Ee, that is equal to the γ-ray energy, Eγ, minus the binding energy of the electron in that orbit. If during ionization the vacancy is created in an inner orbit, a characteristic x-ray or Auger electron will also follow.

Dependence on Z

The photoelectric probability of interaction, τ(atom), also depends strongly on the atomic number of the atom. It is directly proportional to the fourth power of the atomic number, that is, τ(atom) α Z^4. For example, the probability of a γ-ray of a 50-keV interaction with a lead atom (Z = 82) is 11,000 times higher than that with an oxygen atom (Z = 8), because $\frac{[82^4]}{[8^4]} = 11{,}000$.

Of course, if the γ-ray energy happens to be near one of the absorption edges of that atom, this rule is modified.

COMPTON EFFECT

In this process, a high-energy photon is scattered in billiard-ball fashion by an electron, as shown in Figure 6.5. The scattered electron gains energy and the incident photon loses energy. The exact amount of the energy gained by the electron or lost by the photon depends on the angle of scatter and the energy of the incident photon $E\gamma$. In general, though, the larger the angle of scatter for a photon, the more energy it loses to an electron. Thus, the maximum transfer of energy from the photon to the electron occurs when the photon is scattered at an angle of 180° (i.e., back-scattered). The energy of the back-scattered photon (minimum energy of scattered photon) is

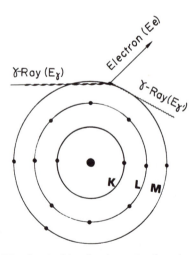

Figure 6.5. Compton interaction. A γ-ray transfers only a partial amount of its energy to an orbital electron (usually the outer shell). The scattered γ-rays carry an energy $E\gamma'$ that is equal to $E\gamma - Ee$, where $E\gamma$ is the energy of the primary γ-ray and Ee is the energy carried by the scattered electron.

Figure 6.6. Energy distribution of the scattered γ-rays and the scattered electrons in a Compton interaction of a 364-keV γ-ray. The maximum amount of energy that a 364-keV γ-ray can transfer to an electron via this process is 210 keV.

related to the energy of the incident photon ($E\gamma$) by the following expression:

$$E\gamma_{minimum} \simeq \frac{E\gamma}{1 + 4\,E\gamma} \quad (E\gamma \text{ is in MeV})$$

For a 1-MeV incident photon, the minimum energy of the scattered photon is 0.200 MeV; for a 0.360 MeV-photon, 0.148 MeV; for a 0.140-MeV photon, 0.090 MeV; and for a 0.080-MeV photon, 0.060 MeV. These values of $E_{minimum}$ are given here as an illustration because of their relevance in γ-ray energy analysis by NaI (Tl) detectors (see Chapter 8). The energies of the scattered photons range from this minimum to that of the incidence photon energy. In Figure 6.6 we show the energy distribution of the scattered photons and scattered electrons for a 360-keV primary photon as a result of Compton interaction.

Dependence on E

The probability of Compton interaction, σ(atom), initially decreases slowly with the increase in energy and then falls off more rapidly.

Dependence on Z

Because each atom contains Z number of electrons, the probability of Compton interaction by an atom, σ(atom), is directly proportional to the atomic number, that is, σ(atom) αZ.

PAIR PRODUCTION

For this interaction to occur, the energy of the γ-ray must be greater than 1.02 MeV. When a γ-

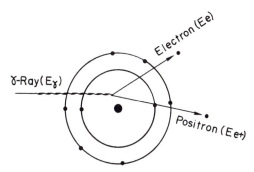

Figure 6.7. Pair production. Under the influence of the positive charge of the nucleus, a γ-ray whose energy, Eγ, is more than 1.02 MeV annihilates and produces a pair of particles (an electron and a positron) that carry the balance of energy, Eγ − 1.02 MeV. The positron is subsequently annihilated in the manner described on p. 52.

ray of energy greater than 1.02 MeV passes through the electric field of a nucleus, it creates an electron and a positron (i.e., part of the γ-ray energy is converted into mass). This process is called pair production and is depicted in Figure 6.7. The excess energy of the γ-ray (Eγ − 1.02 MeV) is shared by e^- and e^+ as kinetic energy.

Dependence on E

The probability of pair production, κ(atom), is zero below 1.02 MeV. At energies higher than 1.02 MeV, κ(atom) increases with increases in E and in fact becomes the dominant mode of interaction above 10 MeV.

Dependence on Z

The probability of pair production, κ(atom), for a given atom varies directly as Z^2.

Dependence of μ(mass) and μ(linear) on Z

So far we have discussed the dependence of μ(atom) on Z for different processes of interaction. How do the linear and mass attenuation coefficients vary with atomic number? The linear attenuation of coefficient, μ(linear), and the mass attenuation coefficient, μ(mass), depends on Z as Z^3, Z^0 (i.e., no dependence on Z), and Z for photoelectric, Compton, and pair production modes of interaction, respectively. In this respect, it is important to remember that when the Compton effect is the dominant mode of interaction, then each gram of any material (i.e., water, iodine, bone, or lead) attenuates the γ- or x-rays to about the same extent. However, atten-

uation per cm^3 of those materials will still differ, in proportion to their density.

Relative Importance of the Three Processes

The total interaction probability of an atom, μ(atom), then, is the sum of the three probabilities, τ(atom), σ(atom), and κ(atom), that is, μ(atom) = τ(atom) + σ(atom) + κ(atom). Because of the complex and varying dependence of μ(atom) on γ-ray energy Eγ and the atomic number Z of the material, generally one of these processes becomes the dominant mode of interaction for a given γ-ray energy and atomic number of the material. Figure 6.8 shows the relative importance of these processes for the 10-keV to 1-MeV energy range for four materials of great importance in nuclear medicine: water (tissue type), bone, sodium iodide [NaI(Tl)], and lead (Pb). In water or bone, most of the interaction of x- or γ-rays above 50 keV is through the Compton effect. For lead, photoelectric interaction is the dominant mode of interaction even up to 1 MeV, although at these energies, Compton interaction does become important. In NaI(Tl), photoelectric effect

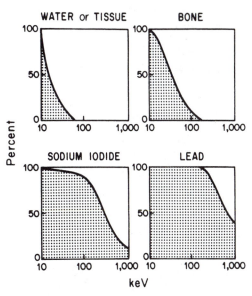

Figure 6.8. Relative contributions of photoelectric and compton interaction to the total attenuation coefficient of water (tissue), bone, sodium iodide, and lead as a function of energy. In water and bone, almost all interactions above 50 keV are via the compton effect, whereas in sodium iodide and lead, the photoelectric effect is the dominant mode of interaction even up to 300 keV. ■, photoelectric; □, Compton effect.

is the dominant mode of interaction up to 300 keV.

INTERACTION OF NEUTRONS

Because neutrons do not have any electric charge, they do not experience the attractive or repulsive forces experienced by charged particles. Instead, these interact in billiard-ball fashion (direct hit) with the nuclei. When the energy of the neutrons is very low, they can easily enter a nucleus and may form radionuclides. Interaction of neutrons does not play a significant role in nuclear medicine, except in the production of some radionuclides by neutron-capture reactions (see Chapter 4), and therefore is not discussed here.

Key Points

1. Charged particles interact with matter through inelastic collisions and have a defined range of penetration, R.

2. Range, R, increases with an increase in energy and decreases with an increase in mass and charge of the particle. It decreases with an increase in density of the interacting material.

3. Linear energy transfer (LET) of a charged particle is an important parameter that affects biological damage.

4. Electrons and positrons interact in identical fashion except that positrons at the end of their range annihilate by combining with an electron. Annihilation produces two γ-rays of 511 keV. These γ-rays travel in opposite direction.

5. Bremsstrahlung is a secondary mechanism of interaction of charged particles. X-rays of various energies are produced when an electron or other charged particle passes in the vicinity of a nucleus.

6. X-rays and γ-rays do not have a well-defined range of interaction. Instead, half-value layer (HVL) is used to define a thickness of a substance that attenuates an x- or γ-ray beam by 50%.

7. For energies of interest in nuclear medicine, three mechanisms, photoelectric (all of the γ-ray energy given to an electron), Compton (γ-ray energy shared between an electron and a scattered γ-ray), and pair production (γ-ray energy is converted into an electron and positron pair) dominate the interaction of x- and γ-rays with matter.

8. Photoelectric effect is the dominant interaction for γ-ray energies up to 500 keV for high-atomic-number materials (>50) such as lead and NaI (Tl).

9. Compton effect dominates in low atomic number materials such as soft tissue and bone above 100 keV.

10. Pair production is important only at high energies (1022 keV and above).

Questions

1. Arrange the following radiations in order of their penetrability: 1-MeV x-ray, 1-MeV electron, 1-MeV α particle, 50-keV characteristic x-ray, and 400-keV γ-ray.

2. List the factors on which the range of a charged particle depends.

3. If you know the range of a charged particle in water, what other information do you need to determine its range in another medium? If you know the linear attenuation coefficient of a γ-ray in water, will the same information let you determine the linear attenuation coefficient of another medium for the same γ-ray?

4. The linear attenuation coefficients of 300-keV γ-rays for tissue, sodium iodide, and lead are approximately 0.12, 0.8, and 4.5 cm^{-1}, respectively. Determine the half-value layer for each material.

5. Photoelectric effect generally decreases sharply with γ-ray energy. In what areas (energies) does this law break down?

6. Determine the energy of a back-scattered γ-ray if the energy of the primary γ-ray is one of the following: 100 keV, 500 keV, or 1 MeV.

7. What are the relationships among the linear attenuation coefficients of ice, water, and steam?

8. The linear attenuation coefficient of bone for a 100-keV γ-rays is 0.2 cm^{-1}. Determine the percentage if 100-keV γ-rays that will pass through a 2-cm-thick bone without any interaction.

9. If in question 8, 80% of the interactions in bone are due to photoelectric effect and 20% due to Compton effect, determine the percentage of 100-keV γ-rays that will interact through photoelectric and Compton interactions, respectively.

10. If a γ-ray interacts through pair production, what is the minimum energy it must have?

Radiation is known to produce a number of deleterious effects in a living system. Therefore, it is important to properly assess the benefits and risks to a patient from a given nuclear medicine procedure, ensuring that the benefits outweigh the risks, if any, by a significant margin. Because one factor that strongly influences the intensity or probability of radiation effects is the energy absorbed by the tissue (radiation dose), this assessment can be performed only if one knows the radiation dose that will be delivered to a patient by a particular procedure. This chapter describes the various methods for determining the radiation dose to a patient from internally administered radionuclides or radiopharmaceuticals. However, in the actual risk estimation, two other important factors, the relative biological effectiveness of the radiation and the tissue sensitivity, are also needed; these are discussed in Chapter 15. Radiation exposure and hazard from external radioactive source are discussed in Chapter 16.

GENERAL COMMENTS ON RADIATION DOSE CALCULATIONS

In nuclear medicine procedures, it is almost impossible to measure the radiation dose directly using any kind of radiation detector. Instead, this has to be calculated by using a variety of physical and biological data and mathematical equations specially developed for this purpose. It should be emphasized, however, at the outset that the accuracy of these calculations is complicated by several factors. First, the physical data needed can be acquired fairly accurately, it is difficult to obtain the biological data needed for these calculations with sufficient accuracy because these are, in practice, extrapolated from animal data or in some cases obtained from limited human data. Second, a variety of assumptions routinely made in these calculations (e.g., uniform distribution, instant uptake of the radiopharmaceutical in the given organ, or single exponential biological elimination) seldom holds true in practice. Third, radiation dose calculations are usually addressed to a hypothetical man known as the "standard man." Various particulars such as the total body weight

and weight of various organs of the standard man are given in Appendix E. These may differ appreciably in an actual case. Finally, the calculated dose is obtained by taking an average over a large volume (greater than 1 cm^3) and therefore cannot be used to estimate radiation dose at cellular level (microdosimetry).

These factors, when combined, make radiation dose calculations susceptible to large errors. Hence, the radiation dose calculations presented here and elsewhere represent an average dose from a given procedure that may vary by a factor of 2, or even more, in an individual case.

DEFINITIONS AND UNITS

Obviously, to calculate the radiation dose, one should know the meaning of radiation dose and radiation dose rate and their units of measurement.

Radiation Dose, D

Radiation dose, or, more precisely, radiation absorbed dose, is a measure of the total energy absorbed from the radiation by 1 g of a substance. Its old unit is the rad, which is a short notation for the radiation absorbed dose. A rad is defined as 100 ergs of absorbed energy per gram of a tissue or substance. If one knows the amount of energy absorbed in erg/g, then to obtain the radiation dose, one divides it by 100 (i.e., 1 rad = 100 erg/g).

In the SI Unit System, rad is replaced by gray (Gy). A gray equals 100 rad or a rad equals 10^{-2} gray. Two commonly used and derived units from gray are centigray (cGy = 10^{-2} Gy = 1 rad) and milligray (mGy = 10^{-3} Gy).

Radiation Dose Rate, $\dfrac{dD}{dt}$

Radiation dose rate, $\dfrac{dD}{dt}$, is defined as the amount of energy absorbed per unit time per gram of tissue. Its units may be expressed in various ways, such as rads (mGy) per minute, rads (cGy) per hour, or rads (Gy) per day.

PARAMETERS OR DATA NEEDED

In a typical situation in nuclear medicine, a known amount of radioactivity of a radiopharmaceutical is administered to a patient. A certain fraction (f) of the radiopharmaceutical is then localized in the organ of interest. One is interested in knowing the radiation dose delivered to this organ and sometimes to various other organs as well. Two types of data are required for these calculations: one related to the decay characteristics of the radionuclide and one to the biological distribution and elimination of the radiopharmaceutical. Table 7.1 lists the various parameters needed for these calculations, together with the units and symbols used here. Some parameters have been defined in Chapters 2 and 3; some are self-evident, and the others are discussed in this chapter. I have retained the old units because a large amount of the data needed in these calculations is still in old units. Its easier to convert the final equations, tables, or results in the SI units, which I have done here at the appropriate places.

CALCULATION OF THE RADIATION DOSE

To calculate the radiation dose, one has to determine the average amount of energy absorbed by 1 g of tissue of a target (organ of interest) from the total energy released by the decay of a given amount of radioactivity. Because x- or γ-rays are more penetrating than particulate radiation, a small x- or γ-ray emitting source, localized at any site in the body, irradiates practically every organ of the body. For example, x- or γ-emitting radionuclide localized only in liver (source S) delivers radiation dose, besides liver, to all other organs (targets T) of the body. Thus, if a radiopharmaceutical is localized in multiple organs (sources), the radiation dose from each source to each organ (targets) has to be calculated before the final determination of the radiation dose to each organ can be made by adding all contributions. The following four steps are involved in the radiation-dose determinations:

1. Calculation of the rate of energy emission (erg/hr) of the various types of radiation emitted by the radionuclide in the source volume.

2. Calculation of the rate of energy absorption from these radiations by the target volume.

3. Calculation of the average dose rate, $\dfrac{dD}{dt}$.

4. Calculation of the average dose D.

This method of radiation dose calculation is known as the absorbed fraction method. The

Table 7.1. Parameters and Symbols Used in the Calculation of Radiation Dose

Parameter	Symbol	Unit
Any given radiation	i	—
Total number of radiations	n	—
Energy of radiation i	E_i	MeV
Frequency of emission of radiation i	n_i	Per decay
Equilibrium dose constant for radiation i	Δ_i	g·rad/μCi·hr
Absorbed fraction	$\phi_i(T \leftarrow S)$	—
Self-absorbed fraction	ϕ_i	—
Target organ	T	—
Source organ	S	—
Mass of target organ	M	g
Radiation dose rate at time t	dD/dt	rad/hr
Radiation dose	D	rad
Radioactivity in source at time t	A(t)	μCi
Radioactive dosage at time 0	A_0	μCi
Fraction localized in the source	f	—
Physical half-life	$T_{\frac{1}{2}}$	hr
Biological half-life	$T_{\frac{1}{2}}(\text{Bio})$	hr
Effective half-life in the source	$T_{\frac{1}{2}}(\text{eff})$	hr

first three steps require mainly physical data such as decay characteristics, organ shape and size, and so on, whereas the fourth step requires biological distribution data.

Step 1: Rate of Energy Emission

Let us first consider a radionuclide that emits only one type of radiation (emission frequency = 1) of energy E (MeV) per decay. One microcurie (3.7×10^4 decay/sec) of this radionuclide will, therefore, emit energy at a rate of $3.7 \times 10^4 \times E$ MeV/sec. If we change the unit of energy from MeV to erg (1 MeV = 1.6×10^{-6} erg) and the unit of time from second to hour (1 hr = 3600 sec), the rate of energy emission by this radionuclide becomes equal to $3.7 \times 10^4 \times 1.6 \times 10^{-6} \times 3600 \times E$ erg/(hr·μCi), or 213E erg/(hr·μCi).

In the case of a radionuclide that emits more than one radiation, say 1, 2, 3 . . . n, with emission frequencies $n_1, n_2, n_3 \ldots n_n$ and energies of $E_1, E_2, E_3 \ldots E_n$, respectively, the rate of energy emission for each type of radiation will be equal to $213n_1E_1$ erg/(hr·μCi) for radiation 1, $213n_2E_2$ erg/(hr·μCi) for radiation 2, and so on.

Step 2: Rate of Energy Absorption

To calculate the rate of absorption of energy by a target volume (T) from a radionuclidic distribution in a source volume (S), we have to define a new quantity known as the absorbed fraction, $\phi_i(T \leftarrow S)$. The absorbed fraction $\phi_i(T \leftarrow S)$ is defined as the ratio of energy absorbed by a target volume (T) from a radiation i to the amount of energy released by a radionuclidic distribution in volume (S) in the form of radiation i. In other words,

$$\phi_i(T \leftarrow S) = \frac{\text{Energy absorbed in volume T from radiation i}}{\text{Energy emitted in volume S as radiation i}}$$

In most problems encountered in nuclear medicine, the radioactivity is distributed within the target volume T itself (i.e., T is the same as S). In that case, the absorbed fraction is known as the self-absorbed fraction and is expressed simply as ϕ_i.

Once $\phi_i(T \leftarrow S)$ is known, the rate of energy absorption by a target volume T is simply obtained by multiplying the rate of energy emission of radiation i (from step 1, $213n_iE_i$) by the absorbed fraction $\phi_i(T \leftarrow S)$, or

Rate of energy absorption by the target volume from radiation i = $213n_iE_i \times \phi_i(T \leftarrow S)$
= $213n_iE_i \phi_i(T \leftarrow S)$ erg/(hr·μCi)

If there are n radiations, the rate of the total energy absorption will be equal to the sum of the energies absorbed from each radiation, that is,
= $213n_1E_1\phi_1(T \leftarrow S) + 213n_2E_2\phi_2(T \leftarrow S) + \ldots$ $213n_nE_n\phi_n(T \leftarrow S)$ erg/(hr·μCi).

The above expression can be written in a concise form as

$$213\sum_{i=1}^{n} n_iE_i\phi_i(T \leftarrow S) \quad \text{erg/(hr·μCi)}$$

where $\sum_{i=1}^{n}$ is the sum of all terms when i changes from 1 to n.

How does one determine $\phi_i(T \leftarrow S)$? Determination of the absorbed fraction requires the exact knowledge of the interaction of radiation with matter, discussed in the previous chapter. Computations of $\phi_i(T \leftarrow S)$ for a number of source and target combinations, from these basic mechanisms of interaction of radiation with matter, are quite involved and require the use of large computers. The *Journal of Nuclear Medicine** published a variety of tables listing $\phi_i(T \leftarrow S)$ for different x- or γ-ray energies and source and target volumes. Table 7.2 lists the absorbed fraction for various organs of a standard man for different x- or γ-ray energies when the radionuclidic distribution is within the same organ (i.e., T is the same as S). For other combinations, the reader is referred to the original articles.*

GENERAL COMMENTS ON $\Phi_i(T \leftarrow S)$

The maximum value of $\phi_i(T \leftarrow S)$ can only be 1. This occurs when all emitted energy is absorbed in the target. The minimum value is 0 and occurs when there is no absorption of energy in the target.

In the case of particulate radiations such as β particles, conversion electrons, or α particles, almost all energy emitted by a radionuclide is absorbed in the volume of distribution itself, provided the source volume is larger than 1 cm³. Then, $\phi_i(T \leftarrow S) = 0$, unless T and S are the same, in which case $\phi_i = 1$. The same holds true for x-

---

* Suppl. No. 1, 1968; Suppl. No. 3, 1969; Suppl. No. 5, 1971.

Table 7.2. Self-Absorbed Fraction ϕ_i for Different γ-Ray Energies and Various Organs

Organ	Energy (keV)						
	15	30	50	100	200	500	1000
Bladder	0.885	0.464	0.201	0.117	0.116	0.116	0.107
Stomach	0.860	0.414	0.176	0.101	0.101	0.101	0.093
Kidneys	0.787	0.298	0.112	0.066	0.068	0.073	0.067
Liver	0.898	0.543	0.278	0.165	0.158	0.157	0.144
Lungs	0.665	0.231	0.089	0.049	0.050	0.051	0.045
Pancreas	0.666	0.195	0.068	0.038	0.042	0.044	0.040
Skeleton	0.893	0.681	0.400	0.173	0.123	0.118	0.110
Spleen	0.817	0.331	0.128	0.071	0.073	0.077	0.070
Thyroid	0.592	0.149	0.048	0.028	0.031	0.032	0.029
Total body	0.933	0.774	0.548	0.370	0.338	0.340	0.321

or γ-radiation with energies less than 10 keV. Thus, these radiations deliver radiation doses only in the volume of distribution and not outside of it.

For x- or γ-radiations with energies higher than 10 keV, the absorbed fraction $\phi_i(T\leftarrow S)$ strongly depends on the energy of the x- or γ-ray; the shape and size of the source volume; and the shape, size, and distance of the target volume. In general, ϕ_i first decreases with an increase in the energy of the x- or γ-ray and then eventually levels off. Notice in Table 7.3 that the absorbed fraction ϕ_i drops sharply with energy up to 100 keV but then does not change significantly from 100 to 500 keV for various organs listed.

Step 3: Dose Rate, $\dfrac{dD}{dt}$

If one now divides the rate of energy absorption by the target with its mass (M), this will give the rate of energy absorption per gram of tissue, which when divided by 100 (to convert erg/g to rad) yields the dose rate for each microcurie of activity, that is, the dose rate,

$$\frac{dD}{dt} = \frac{2.13}{M} \sum_{i=1}^{n} n_i E_i \phi_i(T\leftarrow S) \quad \text{rad/(hr·}\mu\text{Ci)}$$

By defining $\Delta_i = 2.13\, n_i E_i$, this reduces to

$$\frac{dD}{Dt} = \frac{1}{M} \sum_{i=1}^{n} \Delta_i \phi_i(T\leftarrow S) \quad \text{rad/(hr·}\mu\text{Ci)} \quad [1]$$

If the source volume contains A(t) μCi at time t, then the dose rate $\dfrac{dD}{dt}$ from A(t) amount of radioactivity becomes

$$\frac{dD}{dt} = \frac{A(t)}{M} \sum_{i=1}^{n} \Delta_i \phi_i(T\leftarrow S) \quad \text{rad/hr} \quad [2]$$

Step 4: Average Dose, D

The radioactivity A(t) localized in an organ is generally a fraction f of the administered dosage A_0 and is being continuously eliminated, with an effective half-life of $T_{\frac{1}{2}}(\text{eff})$, that is,

$$A(t) = f \cdot A_0 \cdot e^{-\frac{0.693t}{T_{\frac{1}{2}}(\text{eff})}} \quad \mu\text{Ci} \quad [3]$$

Therefore, the dose rate $\dfrac{dD}{dt}$ is continuously decreasing with time and eventually becomes zero. How does one compute the total dose to the patient from the time of administration (t = 0) to the time when the dose rate has finally been reduced to zero? For this, one has to integrate the dose rate $\dfrac{dD}{dt}$ from 0 time to infinite time, or $D = \int_0^\infty \dfrac{dD}{dt} dt$. This involves integration of A(t) that, for a simple case such as equation (3), leads to the following expression:

$$D(T \leftarrow S) =$$
$$1.44 \cdot T_{\frac{1}{2}}(\text{eff}) \cdot \frac{fA_0}{M} \cdot \sum_{n=1}^{n} \Delta_i \cdot \phi_i(T \leftarrow S) \quad \text{rad} \quad [4]$$

In the case where the target and source volume are the same, the self-dose D is given by

$$D = 1.44 \cdot T_{\frac{1}{2}}(\text{eff}) \cdot \frac{fA_0}{M} \cdot \sum_{n=1}^{n} \Delta_i \cdot \phi_i \quad \text{rad} \quad [5]$$

Note that the factor (fA_0/M) in the above

Table 7.3.   S Factors for ^{99m}Tc for Various Sources and Targets (rad/hr·μCi)^{a}

Target	Source									
	Bladder Content	Stomach Content	Kidneys	Liver	Lung	Marrow Red	Bone (Av)	Spleen	Thyroid	Total Body
Bladder wall	1.6×10^{-4}	2.7×10^{-7}	2.8×10^{-7}	1.6×10^{-7}	3.6×10^{-8}	9.9×10^{-7}	5.1×10^{-7}	1.2×10^{-7}	2.1×10^{-9}	2.3×10^{-6}
Bone (total)	9.2×10^{-7}	9.0×10^{-7}	1.4×10^{-6}	1.1×10^{-6}	1.5×10^{-6}	4.0×10^{-6}	1.1×10^{-5}	1.1×10^{-6}	1.0×10^{-6}	2.5×10^{-6}
Stomach wall	2.7×10^{-7}	1.3×10^{-4}	3.6×10^{-6}	1.9×10^{-6}	1.8×10^{-6}	9.5×10^{-7}	5.5×10^{-7}	1.0×10^{-5}	4.5×10^{-8}	2.2×10^{-6}
Kidneys	2.6×10^{-7}	3.5×10^{-6}	1.9×10^{-4}	3.9×10^{-6}	8.4×10^{-7}	2.2×10^{-7}	8.2×10^{-7}	9.1×10^{-6}	3.4×10^{-8}	2.2×10^{-6}
Liver	1.7×10^{-7}	2.0×10^{-6}	3.9×10^{-6}	4.6×10^{-5}	2.5×10^{-6}	9.2×10^{-7}	6.6×10^{-7}	9.8×10^{-7}	9.3×10^{-8}	2.2×10^{-6}
Lungs	2.4×10^{-8}	1.7×10^{-6}	8.5×10^{-7}	2.5×10^{-6}	5.2×10^{-5}	1.2×10^{-6}	9.4×10^{-7}	2.3×10^{-6}	9.4×10^{-7}	2.0×10^{-6}
Marrows	2.2×10^{-6}	1.6×10^{-6}	3.8×10^{-6}	1.6×10^{-6}	1.9×10^{-6}	3.1×10^{-5}	6.6×10^{-6}	1.7×10^{-6}	1.1×10^{-6}	1.1×10^{-6}
Ovaries	7.3×10^{-6}	5.0×10^{-7}	1.1×10^{-6}	4.5×10^{-7}	9.4×10^{-8}	3.2×10^{-6}	8.5×10^{-7}	4.0×10^{-7}	4.9×10^{-9}	2.4×10^{-6}
Spleen	6.6×10^{-7}	1.8×10^{-5}	8.6×10^{-6}	9.2×10^{-7}	2.3×10^{-6}	9.2×10^{-7}	5.8×10^{-7}	3.3×10^{-4}	1.1×10^{-7}	2.2×10^{-6}
Testes	4.7×10^{-6}	5.1×10^{-8}	8.8×10^{-8}	6.2×10^{-8}	7.9×10^{-9}	4.5×10^{-7}	6.4×10^{-7}	4.8×10^{-8}	5.0×10^{-6}	1.7×10^{-6}
Thyroid	2.1×10^{-9}	8.7×10^{-8}	4.8×10^{-8}	1.5×10^{-7}	9.2×10^{-7}	6.8×10^{-7}	7.9×10^{-7}	8.7×10^{-8}	2.3×10^{-3}	1.5×10^{-6}
Total body	1.9×10^{-6}	1.9×10^{-6}	2.2×10^{-6}	2.2×10^{-6}	2.0×10^{-6}	2.2×10^{-6}	6.6×10^{-7}	2.2×10^{-6}	1.8×10^{-6}	2.0×10^{-6}

^{a}To covert to SI unit (Gy/hr·MBq), divide these values by 3.7.

equations is the concentration of the radioactivity in the organ of localization. Therefore, it is the concentration and not the total amount of the radioactivity in an organ that is the primary determinant of the radiation dose.

From these expressions, it is evident *that to minimize the radiation dose to a patient,* smaller amounts of radioactivity (A_0), radiopharmaceuticals with shorter $T_{\frac{1}{2}}$(eff), and radionuclides with smaller absorbed fractions (which means γ-ray energy higher than 100 keV and no particulate emission as discussed earlier; p. 38) are desired.

CUMULATED RADIOACTIVITY

The above equations (4) and (5) assume that the uptake in the organ is instantaneous and the disappearance of the radioactivity from the source can be expressed by a single exponential term, such as in equation (3). This does not have to be so, and often the biokinetics of the radionuclidic distribution is more complex. An example is shown in Figure 7.1. In this case, equation (3) cannot be used to describe the time behavior of the radioactivity in blood or plasma or in organs one and two. For these, the exact time activity curve, $A(t)$, should be used to calculate the cumulated radioactivity $\tilde{A}$, which is defined as $\tilde{A} = \int_0^\infty A(t) \cdot dt$. The unit of $\tilde{A}$ as used here is hr$\cdot\mu$Ci, which means $A(t)$ is measured in μCi and time in hours. Because these calculations are more complicated, we shall not go into the details here.

SIMPLIFICATION OF RADIATION DOSE CALCULATIONS USING "S" FACTOR

Recently, in an attempt to simplify the calculation of radiation dose in routine clinical situations, Snyder and colleagues combined the physical data such as radiations emitted by a radionuclide and the absorbed fractions for various source and target combinations of a standard man into one single term, which they called "S" factor. In fact, S factor is nothing but the dose rate from 1 μCi as given by equation (1). Therefore, S is expressed as follows:

$$S(T \leftarrow S) =$$

$$\frac{dD}{dt} = \frac{1}{M} \sum_{i=1}^{n} \Delta_i \phi_i (T \leftarrow S) \quad \text{rad/(hr} \cdot \mu\text{Ci)} \quad [6]$$

Substitution of S factor in equation (4) simplifies it to the following equation:

$$D(T \leftarrow S) =$$

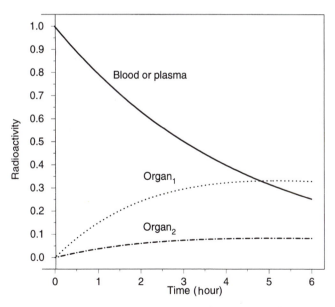

Figure 7.1. Biokinetics of an intravenously administered radiopharmaceutical. Blood or plasma radioactivity decreases with time. A fraction of blood or plasma radioactivity is extracted by organ$_1$ and organ$_2$. Another fraction, not shown here, is excreted. For multicompartmental kinetics such as in this example, none of these curves can be fitted by a monoexponential function given by equation (3). In this case, cumulated activity $\tilde{A}$ needed for radiation dose calculations is determined by either graphic methods or multiexponential curve-fitting methods.

$$1.44 \cdot f \cdot A_0 \cdot T_{\frac{1}{2}}(\text{eff}) \cdot S(T \leftarrow S) \quad \text{rad} \qquad [7]$$

In the case of a radiopharmaceutical with complex biokinetics, such as shown in Figure 7.1, cumulated activity $\tilde{A}$ in each organ should be calculated from the actual biokinetic data. Then,

$$D(T \leftarrow S) = \tilde{A} \cdot S(T \leftarrow S) \quad \text{rad} \qquad [8]$$

S factor depends only on the physical data and is unique for a given radionuclide and a pair of organs of a standard man. Hence, it has to be calculated only once for each radionuclide and each pair of organs (source and target). Snyder and colleagues have calculated these factors for a large number of medically useful radionuclides. These are published as Supplement 11, *Journal of Nuclear Medicine*. Table 7.3 lists some S factors for ^{99m}Tc for a number of organ pairs of a standard man. For other combinations of pairs and radionuclides, the original reference should be consulted. Unit of S factor is rad/(hr·μCi). This can be easily converted into SI units, such as Gy/(hr·MBq), by dividing the S factors given in Table 7.3 with 3.7.

Knowing S factors, the calculation of the radiation dose is simple. One plugs the values of the radioactivity localized in the source organ ($f \cdot A_0$), the effective half-life, ($T_{\frac{1}{2}}(\text{eff})$), and the S factor in equation (7) to obtain the radiation dose.

Caution: The S factor method cannot be applied when the radiation dose is calculated for persons who appreciably differ from a standard man, such as children.

SOME ILLUSTRATIVE EXAMPLES

Problem 1: A liver scan is performed on a patient using 2 mCi of ^{99m}Tc-labeled sulfur colloid. Assuming that 90% of the injected dosage is localized in the liver instantaneously and that the effective half-life, $T_{\frac{1}{2}}(\text{eff})$, is equal to 6 hours, calculate the radiation dose delivered to the liver of the patient using the absorbed fraction method (equation [5]).

Calculation: Because mass of the liver is not given in the problem, we shall assume it to be that of a standard man. Therefore, from Appendix E, M = 1800 g. The initial amount of activity localized in the liver, $A_0(\text{liver}) = 0.90 \times 2000$ μCi = 1800 μCi (66.6 MBq) and $T_{\frac{1}{2}}(\text{eff})$ = 6 hours. Parameters such as n_i, E_i, and Δ_i for ^{99m}Tc and ϕ_i for liver for ^{99m}Tc radiations and the calculations of $\Sigma\Delta_i\phi_i$ are given in Table 7.4. Substituting these values in equation (5) we get

$$\text{Dose (liver)} = (1800/1800) \times 1.44 \times 6 \times$$
$$0.078 = 0.67 \text{ rad} \quad (6.7 \text{ mGy})$$

The remaining 10% of the dosage, if not excreted in a short time from the body, will also contribute a radiation dose to the liver. Its contribution, however, will be small and therefore is ignored here. (Actual calculations will be involved. We will have to construct a table similar to Table 7.4.)

Problem 2: Calculate the radiation dose to the liver, red bone marrow, ovaries, and testes using S factors and the data given in problem 1.

Table 7.4.   Calculation of $\Sigma\Delta_i\phi_i$: Problem 1 (^{99m}Tc)

Radiation i	n_i	E_i	$\Delta_i{}^a$	ϕ_i	$\Delta_i\phi_i$
Gamma 1	—	—	—	—	0
Conversion electron	0.986	0.002	0.004	1	0.004
Gamma 2	0.883	0.140	0.264	0.16	0.042
K-conversion electron	0.088	0.119	0.022	1	0.022
L-conversion electron	0.011	0.138	0.003	1	0.003
M-conversion electron	0.004	0.140	0.001	1	0.001
Gamma 3					
Conversion electron	0.01	0.122	0.003	1	0.003
K (α) x-ray	0.064	0.018	0.003	0.88	0.0026
K (β) x-ray	0.012	0.021	—	0.87	—
KLL Auger electron	0.015	0.015	—	1	—
LMM Auger electron	0.106	0.002	—	1	—
MXY Auger electron	1.23	0.0004	—	1	—
			$\Sigma\Delta_i\phi i = 0.078^b$		

$^a\Delta_i = 2.13 n_i E_i$.
^{b}Sum of all $\Delta_i\phi_i$.

Calculation: As in problem 1, $T_{\frac{1}{2}}(\text{eff}) = 6$ hours, $A_0(\text{liver}) = 1800\ \mu\text{Ci}$ (66.6 MBq), and from Table 7.3,

$$S(\text{liver} \leftarrow \text{liver}) = 4.6 \times 10^{-5}$$
$$S(\text{marrow} \leftarrow \text{liver}) = 1.6 \times 10^{-6}$$
$$S(\text{ovaries} \leftarrow \text{liver}) = 4.5 \times 10^{-7}$$
$$S(\text{testes} \leftarrow \text{liver}) = 6.2 \times 10^{-8}$$

Substituting these values in equation (7), we get

$$D(\text{liver} \leftarrow \text{liver}) = 1.44 \times 1800 \times 6 \times 4.6 \times 10^{-5} = 0.72\ \text{rad}\quad (7.2\ \text{mGy})$$
$$D(\text{marrow} \leftarrow \text{liver}) = 1.44 \times 1800 \times 6 \times 1.6 \times 10^{-6} = 0.025\ \text{rad}\quad (0.25\ \text{mGy})$$
$$D(\text{ovaries} \leftarrow \text{liver}) = 1.44 \times 1800 \times 6 \times 4.5 \times 10^{-7} = 0.007\ \text{rad}\quad (0.07\ \text{mGy})$$
$$D(\text{testes} \leftarrow \text{liver}) = 1.44 \times 1800 \times 6 \times 6.2 \times 10^{-8} = 0.001\ \text{rad}\quad (0.01\ \text{mGy})$$

This problem illustrates the simplicity of the S factor approach in the calculation of the radiation dose. Without constructing tables like Table 7.4, one is able to calculate radiation doses easily, not for one but several organs. Again we have neglected the contribution to the radiation dose of the 10% radiopharmaceutical dosage not localized in the liver. However, calculation of the radiation doses from this fraction will also be straightfor-

ward provided one knows the organ of localization and the effective half-life. Also note that the dose to the liver by this method is slightly higher than that in problem 1. This in part is due to the fact that standard man data used for the calculation of S factors are slightly different than that used to compute the original absorbed fractions, ϕ_i.

Problem 3: A patient is treated for hyperthyroidism with 5 mCi of ^{131}I. Calculate the radiation dose to the thyroid of the patient, assuming that the weight of the thyroid gland is 30 g, the effective half-life is 4 days, and the measured thyroid uptake is 45%.

Calculation: Because the thyroid mass (30 g) is quite different from the thyroid mass (20 g) of the standard man (Appendix E), we cannot use the S factor method here. Thyroid mass M = 30 g. The initial amount of activity localized in the thyroid, $A_0(\text{thyroid}) = 0.45 \times 5000\ \mu\text{Ci} = 2250\ \mu\text{Ci}$ (83.25 MBq), and $T_{\frac{1}{2}}(\text{eff}) = 4\ \text{days} = 4 \times 24\ \text{hours} = 96\ \text{hours}$. Parameters such as n_i, E_i, and Δ_i for ^{131}I; ϕ_i for thyroid for ^{131}I radiations; and the calculations of $\Sigma\Delta_i\phi_i$ are given in Table 7.5. Substituting these values in equation (5),

$$D(\text{thyroid}) = (2250/30) \times 1.44 \times 96 \times 0.433$$
$$\text{rad} = 4489\ \text{rad}\quad (44.89\ \text{Gy})$$

The important thing to note here is that if we

Table 7.5. Calculation of $\Sigma\Delta_i\phi_i$: Problem 3 (^{131}I)

Radiation i	n_i	E_i	Δ_i	ϕ_i	$\Delta_i\phi_i$
Beta 1	0.016	0.070	0.002	1	0.002
Beta 2	0.069	0.095	0.014	1	0.014
Beta 3	0.005	0.143	0.001	1	0.001
Beta 4	0.905	0.192	0.369	1	0.369
Beta 5	0.006	0.286	0.004	1	0.004
Gamma 1	0.017	0.080	0.003	0.035	—
K-conversion electron	0.029	0.046	0.003	1	0.003
Gamma 2					
Conversion electron	0.004	0.129	0.001	1	0.001
Gamma 3	0.047	0.284	0.029	0.03	0.001
K-conversion electron	0.002	0.250	0.001	1	0.001
Gamma 4	0.002	0.326	0.001	0.03	—
Gamma 5	0.833	0.364	0.646	0.03	0.019
K-conversion electron	0.017	0.330	0.012	1	0.012
L-conversion electron	0.003	0.359	0.002	1	0.002
Gamma 6	0.003	0.503	0.003	0.03	—
Gamma 7	0.069	0.637	0.093	0.03	0.003
Gamma 8	0.016	0.723	0.025	0.03	0.001
K (α) x-rays	0.038	0.030	0.002	0.15	—
			$\Sigma\Delta_i\phi_i = 0.433^a$		

^{a}Sum of all $\Delta_i\phi_i$.

had used only the particulate radiations of ^{131}I in our calculations (Table 7.5), the radiation dose would have been 4043 rad (i.e., 90% of the radiation dose to the thyroid by ^{131}I is delivered by particulate [mainly β^-] radiations). This is the reason why ^{131}I is a good radionuclide for use in therapy and not diagnosis.

RADIATION DOSES IN ROUTINE IMAGING PROCEDURES

Table 7.6 lists the average radiation doses delivered to an adult patient from a number of radiopharmaceuticals commonly used in nuclear medicine. Although an internally administered radiopharmaceutical delivers a radiation dose to practically each and every organ in the body, only the total body and critical organ (the one that receives the highest radiation dose) radiation doses are used to illustrate the extent of the radiation doses routinely delivered to the pa-

tients. Their significance in terms of the risk involved is discussed in Chapter 15.

In children, the radiopharmaceutical dosage is proportionally reduced to account for the smaller surface area or weight of a child as compared with an adult. As a result, similar concentrations (radioactivity/g) are localized in both cases. Still, because of the smaller size of organs, the radiation doses in children will be slightly different (some higher and some lower) from the adult radiation doses.

Radiation Dose to a Fetus

Because a fetus is more sensitive to radiation than an adult, it is not generally advisable to administer radiopharmaceuticals to a pregnant patient. However, there are occasions when, either because of strong medical reasons or inadvertently, a pregnant patient may receive radiopharmaceuticals. In these cases, it is essential to

Table 7.6.   Radiation Doses in Common Imaging Procedures

Radiopharmaceutical	Radioactivity Dosage		Radiation Dose (Total Body)		Radiation Dose (Critical Organ)		Critical Organ
	mCi	MBq	rad	mGy	rad	mGy	
^{99m}Tc-labeled	10	370	0.15	1.5	2.5	25	Stomach
Pertechnetate							
Glucoheptonate	20	740	0.15	1.5	4.5	45	Bladder
Phosphate, etc.	10	370	0.1	1	1.5	15	Bladder
Sulfur Colloid	3	111	0.05	0.5	0.9	9	Liver
MA albumin	3	111	0.05	0.5	1	10	Lungs
DMSA	6	222	0.1	1	4.0	40	Kidneys
DTPA	20	740	0.1	1.2	3.5	35	Bladder
Red cells	20	740	0.4	4	0.4	4	Total body
Iron ascorbate	2	74	0.01	0.1	1	10	Kidneys
HIDA, etc.	5	185	0.05	0.5	1.6	16	Small intestine
Mertiatide (MAG3)	10	370	0.07	0.7	4.8	48	Bladder
Sestamibi (Cardiolite)	30	1110	0.5	5	5.4	54	Upper large intestine
Teboroxime (Cardiotec)	20	740	0.3	3	2.5	25	Upper large intestine
Tetrofosmin (Myoview)	30	1110	0.4	4	3.6	36	Gallbladder wall
Exametazime (Ceretec)	20	740	0.3	3	5.2	52	Lacrimal glands
^{67}Ga Citrate	5	185	1.3	13	4.5	45	Lower large intestine
^{111}In-DTPA	0.5	18.5	0.04	0.4	2.0	20	Spinal chord
(Cisternography)							
^{111}In-Pentetreotide (OctreoScan)	3	111	0.5	5	74	7.4	Spleen
^{131}I-Iodide	0.05	1.85	0.2	2	75	750	Thyroid
^{123}I-Iodide	0.1	3.7	0.004	0.04	2.2	22	Thyroid
^{123}I-Iofetamine (SPECTamine)	6	222	0.5	5	4.7	47	Retina
^{131}I-Iodohippurate	0.2	7.4	0.006	0.06	0.2	2	Kidneys
^{133}Xe	10	370	0.001	0.01	0.3	3	Lungs
^{201}Tl-Thallous Chloride	3	111	0.7	7	4.5	45	Kidneys

DMSA, 2, 3-dimercaptosuccinic acid; DTPA, diethylenetriamine pentaacetic acid; and HIDA, (2,6-dimethylacetanilide)iminodiacetic acid.

estimate the radiation dose to the fetus. The radiation dose to the fetus in these circumstances is derived from two sources: the radionuclide distributed in the mother's body and the radionuclide distributed in the fetal body due to the placental crossover. For most ^{99m}Tc-labeled radiopharmaceuticals (except pertechnetate), there is little placental crossover, and therefore most of the radiation dose is derived from distribution in the mother's body. In these cases, the estimated radiation dose to the fetus is between 200 and 400 mrad (2–4 mGy) from 10 mCi (370 MBq) of the administered radioactivity.

Radionuclides such as ^{131}I, ^{67}Ga, and ^{201}Tl, cross the placenta and therefore, depending on the stage of pregnancy, can deliver a relatively large radiation dose. In early pregnancy (first trimester) when the placental crossover is small, the radiation dose to the fetus from diagnostic dosages of these radionuclides is under 1 rad (10 mGy).

Key Points

1. Radiation absorbed dose is an important physical parameter that determines biological effect.

2. It is defined as 100 ergs of energy absorbed by 1 g of tissue and its unit is rad. The SI unit is gray and it equals 100 rad.

3. Calculation of radiation dose involves four steps: rate of energy emission, rate of energy absorption, dose rate, and dose.

4. Radiation dose increases with an increase in dosage of the radiopharmaceutical and effective half-life in the tissue. It also depends on the mass of the tissue and the energies of radiations emitted by the radionuclide.

5. Routine radiopharmaceuticals deliver radiation doses under 1 rad (0.01 Gy) to the total body and under 10 rad (0.1 Gy) to the critical organ.

Questions

1. Convert the following radiation doses into SI units: (a) 350 rad, (b) 120 mrad, (c) 5 rad.

2. List the major factors on which the radiation dose from a radiopharmaceutical depends.

3. What is the largest source of error in the radiation dose calculations?

4. A β emitter is distributed with uniform concentration in (a) a sphere, (b) a cylinder, and (c) a cube of the same volume. Is the radiation dose the same or different in the three cases?

5. What if the radionuclide in problem 2 is a pure γ emitter?

6. On what factors does the absorbed fraction, ϕ_i, depend?

7. For a monoexponential decay (equation [3]), what is the relationship between the cumulated radioactivity, $\tilde{A}$, and f, A_0, and $T_{\frac{1}{2}}(\text{eff})$.

8. How does the S factor simplify the radiation dose calculations? What are its limitations? Can this method be used to calculate a radiation dose for a given patient?

9. A γ emitter is localized in a patient's liver. Can it deliver a radiation dose to his or her brain, thyroid, lungs, spleen, testes, or ovaries? If yes, which of these organs will receive the maximum and minimum dose?

10. What nuclear medicine procedure delivers the largest radiation dose to the total body?

When high-energy radiation interacts with matter, it produces certain physical or chemical changes in matter. These changes, which can be either transitory or permanent, are the basis for detection of high-energy radiation (referred to as radiation, for conciseness, in this chapter). However, these changes generally are too minute to be directly detected by our senses. Therefore, highly complex methods have been developed to detect radiation. Here I describe the various detectors used in nuclear medicine. However, two relevant questions, what properties of radiation and what properties of detectors are important in nuclear medicine, are addressed first.

WHAT DO WE WANT TO KNOW ABOUT RADIATION?

Basically, we are interested in knowing one or more of the following.

Simple Detection

Is radiation present? This question usually does not arise in nuclear medicine because one always administers a known radionuclide to the patient. In special circumstances, however, such as contamination of surroundings or personnel, one may be faced with this question. Of course, any presence of radiation will lead to the next question.

Quantity of Radiation

How much radiation or radioactivity is present? In any use of radiation in nuclear medicine, one must answer this basic question, if not in absolute terms, then in relative terms (i.e., with respect to a standard). In dynamic studies, this question is modified as how much radiation or radioactivity is present at a given time? This requires measurement of radioactivity or counting rate as a function of time.

Energy of the Radiation

In nuclear medicine, unlike nuclear physics, one is not interested in knowing the energy of the radiation per se. From practical considerations, however, it is helpful in two ways: to discriminate against undesired events such as scattered γ-rays that may be identified by energy measurement and to identify two radionuclides that may be used simultaneously.

Nature of Radiation

In general, in nuclear medicine one knows the kind of radiation with which one is involved. However, again in cases of contamination, one may be faced with the task of identifying the type of the radiation.

Not every detector can answer all of these questions. One type of detector can measure each radiation interacting with it individually but not the energy of the radiation (e.g., Geiger-Mueller [GM] counters). Scintillator detectors can measure both the energy and the individual interaction of the radiation. Ionization chambers cannot be used as counters or to measure energy of radiation but are still useful under many circumstances, such as measurement of radiation "exposure." Exposure depends on both the energies and the number of radiations interacting in the detector and is a useful concept in radiation protection from external x- or γ-emitting radiation sources (see Chapter 16).

WHAT MAKES ONE RADIATION DETECTOR BETTER THAN ANOTHER?

The answer to this complex question primarily depends on the use one wishes to make of the radiation detector. However, the following properties of a detector are of significance in radionuclidic imaging, which is the primary activity in nuclear medicine.

Intrinsic Efficiency or Sensitivity

Intrinsic efficiency (E_i) of a detector is the measure of its ability to detect radiation and is generally defined as the ratio of the number of rays of a given radiation (α, β, or γ) detected to the number of rays incident on the sensitive volume of the detector:

$$E_i = \frac{\text{Number of rays detected by the detector}}{\text{Number of rays incident on the sensitive volume of the detector}}$$

A value of 0.5 (50%) for the intrinsic efficiency means that only one-half of the rays incident on the sensitive volume of the detector is detected and the other half does not interact within the sensitive volume. The higher the intrinsic efficiency of a detector, the better it is for use in nuclear medicine. Higher intrinsic efficiency allows a shortened imaging time, a reduced radiation dose to patients, or both. Intrinsic efficiency of a detector primarily depends on the linear-attenuation coefficient, μ(linear), and the thickness of the sensitive volume.

Dead Time or Resolving Time

Dead time or resolving time (used interchangeably here) is a measure of the ability of a detector to function accurately at high count rates encountered when large amounts of radioactivities are used. For any detector, there is a small but finite interval between the time when a ray interacts with a detector and the time when the detector responds and the event is recorded. This interval is known as "dead time" or resolving time of the detector. What happens if a second ray arrives and starts interacting with the detector while it is still processing the first ray? The response of a detector under such circumstance is broadly described under two categories: paralyzable and nonparalyzable. Both mechanisms may be operative in the same detector.

In the paralyzable situation when the second ray arrives within the dead time of the detector, the detector becomes insensitive for another time interval equal to the time of arrival of the second ray. For example, if the dead time of a detector is 100 μsec and the second ray arrives after 30 μsec of the arrival of the first, the detector becomes insensitive for a total of 30 + 100 = 130 μsec, provided, of course, no third ray arrives within this interval. In that case, the interval will be extended further depending on the time of arrival of the third ray and so on. Thus, depending on the count rate, which determines the average time interval between the arrival of two successive rays, in the paralyzable case a large number of rays can be lost without registering in the detector.

In the nonparalyzable case, the insensitive period of the detector is not affected by the arrival of the second ray. The second ray or others arriving in this insensitive period are lost. Figure 8.1 shows the effect of dead time on various count rates for a paralyzable and nonparalyzable detector. For a nonparalyzable detector, the detector response (observed count rate) at first increases linearly with the true count rate but then reaches a plateau. On the other hand, for a paralyzable detector, the initial part of the response is the same, but after reaching a peak, the observed count rate actually starts decreasing with an increase in the true count rate. In other words, for paralyzable-type counters, the same observed count rate is obtained with two different true count rates (or radioactivities), one low and one high; this is a serious pitfall to be aware of.

Ideally, the detector should have as short a dead time as possible because it will detect very high count rates without significant losses. However, for the count rates encountered in nuclear medicine from the routine dosage of the current radiopharmaceuticals, a system dead time of about 10 μsec is acceptable. However, for fast dynamic imaging of the heart where higher count rates are desirable, system dead time shorter than 10 μsec (2–3 μsec) are essential.

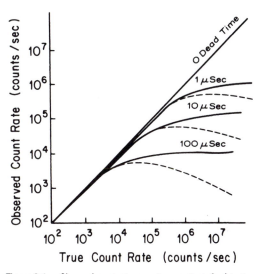

Figure 8.1. Observed count rate versus true count rate for detectors with different dead times. Solid lines, nonparalyzable detectors; broken lines, paralyzable detectors. If both components, paralyzable and nonparalyzable, contribute to the dead time, the response will be in between the two extremes. Note that as the dead time of a detector increases, the usable count-rate range (linear portion) becomes smaller.

Energy Discrimination Capability or Energy Resolution

The ability of a detector to distinguish between two radiations of different energies (e.g., two γ-rays of different energies) is known as its energy discrimination capability or energy resolution. Full width at half maximum (FWHM), which is commonly used as a measure of energy resolution and is defined later in this chapter, represents the minimum difference necessary between the energies of two γ-rays if they are to be identified as having different energies. If the FWHM of a detector is 20 keV, then two γ-rays with a difference in energy less than 20 keV cannot be distinguished by this detector. A lower value of FWHM indicates a better energy discrimination capability. Another way to look at FWHM is to consider it as a measure of error in the energy determination of an x- or γ-ray by a detector. The lower this error is, the more accurate the detector will be in measuring γ-ray energy and therefore in detecting small changes in the energy of x- or γ-rays.

Other Considerations

Because most detectors use electronic components whose behavior quite often is susceptible to change with fluctuations in line voltage and environment temperature, detectors whose response is not appreciably affected by these fluctuations are preferred. Detectors should also be portable (depending on their desired use), simple to operate, and, of course, inexpensive.

TYPES OF DETECTORS

With this background in mind, various types of radiation detectors are discussed: gas-filled detectors, scintillation detectors, and semiconductor detectors. Their main characteristics and uses are summarized in Table 8.1.

Gas-Filled Detectors

As discussed in Chapter 6, the first action of high-energy radiation on matter is the production of ionization. In general, it is not possible to measure the amount of ionization produced in matter except in gases and some solids, known as semiconductors. The measurement of the amount of ionization produced by radiation in a small gas volume is the basis of three types (i.e., ionization chambers, proportional counters, and GM counters) of gas-filled detectors.

MECHANISM OF GAS-FILLED DETECTORS

To explain the mechanism of detection of gas-filled detectors, let us consider what happens when ionization is produced by a ray or particle in a gas volume enclosed between two electrodes with an applied voltage V (Fig. 8.2). When the applied voltage, V, between the two electrodes is zero, the ion pairs produced by the radiation recombine to form neutral atoms or molecules, and no current flows in the circuit. However, under the influence of the electric field that exists between the two electrodes when V is greater than zero, some ion pairs reach the electrodes and a transient current is produced in the circuit. The amount of current produced depends on several factors, such as the applied voltage V; distance between the two electrodes; type of gas; volume, pressure, and temperature of the gas; and geometry and shape of the electrodes. The most important parameter, however, is the applied voltage, V, between the two electrodes. The

Table 8.1.   Some Characteristics of Common γ-Ray Detectors

Detector	Intrinsic Efficiency	Dead Time	Energy Discrimination	Uses in Nuclear Medicine
Ionization chambers	Very low	—[a]	None	Dose calibrators
Proportional counters	Very low	$\sim$ msec	Moderate	Rarely used
Geiger-Mueller counters	Moderate	$\sim$ msec	None	Radiation survey work
NaI (T1) scintillation counters	High	$\sim$ μsec	Moderate	Most widely used detector, well counters, scintillation camera
Semiconductor Ge (Li) counters	Moderate	<1 μsec	Very good	Neutron activation analyses

[a]Cannot be used as a counter.

Figure 8.2. Schematic of gas-filled radiation detector. The two electrodes collect the ion pairs produced in the gas by radiation.

amount of the current produced by a single radiation in a typical gas-filled detector as a function of voltage, V, is shown in Figure 8.3. The dependence of the current on voltage is complex. There are five distinct regions that need explanation. Keep in mind that if no ionization is produced by the radiation in the gas volume, the current will be zero irrespective of the voltage applied.

Region I or Recombination

The voltage is low so that some ion pairs produced by a ray or particle (called primary ion pairs) are still able to recombine and form neutral atoms or molecules. In other words, there is an incomplete collection of the primary ion pairs

by the electrodes. As the voltage increases, more primary ion pairs are collected by the electrodes and more current flows.

Region II or Ionization Plateau   *Ion saturation*

The voltage is now sufficiently high to attract all primary ion pairs produced by a ray or particle to the electrodes, and there is little recombination. The amount of the current does not change appreciably with an increase in the voltage because all primary ion pairs produced by the radiation have been collected. The amount of current produced by a single ray or particle (total number of primary ion pairs) is still small and cannot be detected unless integrated for interaction of many rays or particles.

Region III or Proportional Region   *Gas Amplification*

The voltage is even higher. This is not only enough to attract all primary ion pairs to the electrodes but is also sufficient to provide enough energy to some primary ion pairs that now produce secondary ion pairs through collisions with neutral atoms and molecules of the gas. The amount of secondary ion pairs produced depends on the energy acquired by the primary ion pairs, which depends on the voltage. As a result, the amount of current produced by a radiation increases with increase in voltage.

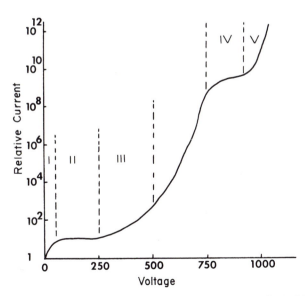

Figure 8.3. Plot of current as a function of voltage (V) applied to the two electrodes of Figure 8.2. Origin of the five regions marked I, II, III, IV, and V is explained in the text. Region I, ion-pair recombination; region II, ionization chambers operate in this region; region III, proportional counters; region IV, Geiger-Mueller counters. The unmarked region between regions III and IV is of no practical importance.

The current is now sufficiently high for detection in response to a single ray or particle interaction in the gas volume. It is also proportional to the energy of the radiation. However, as the voltage increases further (unmarked region between III and IV), this relationship with energy becomes nonlinear.

Region IV or GM Plateau

The voltage is so much higher that the primary ion pairs produced by a ray or particle acquire large energy to produce a large number of secondary ion pairs and excitations, which then strike the metallic electrodes and more neutral gas molecules to produce more ionizations and excitations. The de-excitation of the molecules produces ultraviolet light, which produces more ionization. The result is that the total gas volume is in a temporary state of discharge and the amount of current produced is more or less independent of the voltage and the energy of the radiation.

Region V   *Spontaneous Gas ionization*

The voltage is so high that radiation is not necessary to produce discharge. Under the influence of such a high electric field, the electrons are pulled out from the atomic shells, the atoms and molecules become ionized, and a discharge may be established even without radiation.

IONIZATION DETECTOR (CHAMBER)

Ionization detectors are one of the earliest types of gas-filled detectors used for radiation measurement. The operating voltage in these detectors lies in region II of Figure 8.3. In this region, small fluctuations in the applied voltage do not affect the current significantly. As a result,

ionization chambers are highly stable and reliable. These can be made in a variety of shapes and sizes and are relatively inexpensive. Their main disadvantages are a poor intrinsic efficiency for x- or γ-rays and a lack of energy discrimination. Because the amount of current produced in response to a single ray or particle is small, these cannot be used as counters. Therefore, their principal use is in the measurement of radiation exposure such as that encountered in diagnostic and therapeutic radiology. They are principally used in nuclear medicine as "dose calibrators" to measure radioactivity in the microcurie-to-curie range. Occasionally, these may be used to measure exposure to individual radiation workers in the form of "pocket dosimeters," as discussed in chapter 16.

Dose Calibrator

Dose calibrators are, generally, cylindrically shaped ionization chambers filled with a rare gas such as argon at high pressure (~20 atmospheres). High pressure increases the density of the gas, which increases the intrinsic efficiency of the ionization chamber. There is a small hole along the axis of the cylinder so that the radioactive sample whose radioactivity is to be measured can be inserted close to the center of the ionization chamber (Fig. 8.4). This type of geometric arrangement increases the overall sensitivity of a detector and is known as 4π arrangement (see Chapter 9). The outside walls of the chamber are appropriately shielded to minimize the interference from radioactive sources outside the chamber.

The principle and operation of a dose calibrator are simple. The current produced in the ionization chamber by a given radioactive source

Figure 8.4.   A simplified schematic of a "dose calibrator."

in a given geometric arrangement is directly proportional to the amount of the radioactivity of the source. However, different radionuclides with the same amount of radioactivity produce different amounts of current. This difference in current produced by the same radioactivities of different radionuclides arises mainly from the differences in emission frequency n_i and the energy E_i of γ-rays emitted by them. Therefore, before an ionization chamber can be used as a dose calibrator, it needs to be calibrated for the desired radionuclides individually. The initial calibration is performed by measuring the amount of current produced for 1 mCi of a given radionuclide. This process is repeated for all desired radionuclides. Sources of known radioactivity (to a 5% or less accuracy) can be obtained from the National Bureau of Standards, who determine the radioactivity of these sources accurately by complex and time-consuming methods. Once the calibration factors are known, the unknown radioactivity of a given radionuclide is easily obtained by dividing the current produced by the unknown radioactivity with the calibration factor for that radionuclide.

In commercial dose calibrators (Fig. 8.4), the ionization chamber is connected to a digital current meter and the calibration factors for a number of radionuclides are predetermined and stored so the results of the unknown radioactivity are directly displayed in microcurie, millicurie, or curie (or MBq, etc.) when the appropriate button for the given radionuclide is selected. With these calibrators, however, it should be remembered that when we press a button labeled "^{99m}Tc," all we are doing is recalling the calibration factor of ^{99m}Tc. We are not discriminating against other radionuclides. A ^{99m}Tc source in a dose calibrator will display radioactivity at other radionuclidic settings, but these will not be correct radioactivity of ^{99m}Tc sample. As a result, dose calibrators cannot be used to determine the radioactivity of a mixed (containing more than one radionuclide) sample except as described under ^{99}Mo Breakthrough Measurement, below.

Quality Assurance.   To ensure the proper operation of a dose calibrator, its linearity (i.e., the current is proportional to the radioactivity for a given radionuclide) and accuracy should be measured yearly. Accuracy should be better than

10%. For routine assurance, a constancy check should be performed daily by measuring the radioactivity of a standard source consisting of long-lived radionuclide such as ^{137}Cs or ^{57}Co. The measured radioactivity should not vary more than 10% from the radioactivity of the standard source, corrected for the decay. It must also be noted that the calibration factors are valid only for a given geometric setup, source volume, and source container. If the shape or type of the source container or the volume of the source is changed appreciably, the calibration factor will change and therefore should be measured again.

^{99}Mo Breakthrough Measurement.   Although a dose calibrator cannot measure accurately the radioactivities of two radionuclides when present simultaneously in a sample, it can be used to measure the radioactivity of ^{99}Mo breakthrough in the ^{99m}Tc eluate obtained from a generator by using an ingenious method. It involves the use of a lead container of a wall thickness sufficient to attenuate essentially all γ-rays (140 keV) emanating from a typical ^{99m}Tc radioactivity obtained from a generator. This thickness of lead is not enough to attenuate high-energy ^{99}Mo γ-rays (740 and 778 keV) to any great extent. Lead containers of appropriate thickness are usually provided by the manufactures of dose calibrators. To measure ^{99}Mo breakthrough, two measurements are made on the vial containing ^{99m}Tc eluate: on the ^{99m}Tc setting without the lead container, which gives the ^{99m}Tc radioactivity, and at the ^{99}Mo setting with the vial in the lead container, which, when multiplied by the attenuation factor for ^{99}Mo γ-rays (provided by the manufacturer), yields the ^{99}Mo radioactivity. Because the ^{99m}Tc radioactivity in the eluate is typically 1000 times the ^{99}Mo radioactivity (parent breakthrough), error in the ^{99m}Tc radioactivity in the presence of small amount of ^{99}Mo radioactivity is small and therefore neglected. Division of the ^{99}Mo radioactivity (in microcurie) by the ^{99m}Tc radioactivity (in millicurie) yields the ^{99}Mo breakthrough in the appropriate unit.

PROPORTIONAL DETECTOR (COUNTER)

These detectors operate in region III of Figure 8.3, where there is a built-in amplification ($\sim 10^6$) of the primary ionization through the production of secondary ionization. A sufficient amount of current is produced by a single ray for it to be counted, and the current is directly proportional to the energy of the radiation. Hence, a proportional detector, unlike the ionization chamber, can be used to count individual events and to determine the energy of the radiation. Proportional counters require a sufficient amount of expertise in their construction and use. Their stability, with time and voltage fluctuations, is not as good as of the ionization chambers. Proportional counters are rarely used in nuclear medicine.

GEIGER-MUELLER DETECTOR (COUNTER)

The operating voltage of GM detectors is in the region IV of Figure 8.3. The incoming particle in this case causes a discharge in the gas, and the amount of the current produced is more or less independent of the energy of the radiation and of the voltage. Once the discharge is established in the gas by a ray, how does one stop the process so that the detector is ready for the next ray? This is accomplished chemically. Small amounts of halogens or their organic compounds are introduced in the gas as impurities. These impurities, known as chemical quenchers, absorb the ultraviolet light produced during the discharge and the energy from the secondary ion pairs. Absorption of energy by the quencher molecules causes the discharge to stop but leads to their dissociation. However, within a short time, most quencher molecules are able to recombine to form the original molecule. Therefore, there is little depletion of the quencher. It takes from about 50 to 200 μsec to quench the discharge. During this time, the GM counter does not respond to another radiation; therefore, this is approximately the dead time of the detector and is nonparalyzable. The maximum usable count rate for a typical GM counter is 60,000 counts/min.

GM detectors are the most sensitive of the gas-filled detectors. They can be made in any shape and size, are easy to operate, and are quite stable in reference to temperature and voltage fluctuations; however, they cannot measure the energy of a radiation. For the detection of β-rays, there is a small window made of thin aluminized Mylar either at the end or one side of the GM tube. For the detection of x- or γ-rays, this window is generally closed. Also, because the interaction of x- or γ-rays in the gas volume itself is minimal, the detection of these radiations is primarily through the photo- and Compton-electrons generated in the inner walls of the GM tube. These are rugged, portable, and comparatively inexpensive detectors. The principal use of GM detectors in nuclear medicine is in radiation protection work for surveying the contamination of surroundings and personnel from x- and γ-ray emitting radionuclides.

Scintillation Detectors (Counters)

A variety of substances known as phosphors scintillate (produce light) under the influence of high-energy radiation. This property is used for the detection of radiation by instruments known as scintillation detectors. However, for the detection of the light generated in a material, it should be able to be transmitted out of the material itself. In liquids, it poses no serious problem. For solids, only single crystals or glasses can be used because in powders (microcrystals), light is absorbed and scattered at the boundaries of the microcrystals, thereby causing significant and variable loss of light before its detection.

Two other types of substances, thermoluminescent and photoluminescent, are also used as radiation detectors. These substances do not produce light immediately after interacting with radiation but can store some of the energy given by the radiation for a long time. The stored energy is released in the form of light at a later time by either heating (thermoluminescent) the irradiated substance or exposing it to laser light (photoluminescent). Thermoluminescent detectors are used in radiation monitoring and are discussed in Chapter 16. Photoluminescent detectors have not found use in nuclear medicine but are finding uses in diagnostic radiology, particularly in digital radiology.

A typical scintillation counter is shown schematically in Figure 8.5. It consists of a scintillator, photomultiplier (PM) tube to detect the light, preamplifier, amplifier, and assorted electronics such as pulse-height selector and a count-rate meter or scaler for automatic data collection and analysis. The following section outlines the mechanism of a typical scintillation counter used in the detection of γ-rays. Liquid scintillation counters used in the detection of high-energy charged particles (i.e., α and β) are described in Chapter 9.

Figure 8.5. Schematic of a scintillation counter. The four controls denoted by HV (high voltage), G (gain of the amplifier), LL or E (lower level or energy), and W or ΔE (window width or energy width) are important in the operation of a scintillation counter. In the PM tube, C stands for photocathode, FE for focusing electrode, and A for anode.

SCINTILLATOR

The number of scintillating substances (scintillators) is large. Anthracene, naphthalene, various plastics, alkali halide crystals doped with or without impurities such as NaI(Tl) or CsF, lead tungstate, bismuth germanate, and aromatic compounds such as terphenyl and 2,5-diphenyloxazole have all been used as scintillators.

Mechanism of Light Production

Because the mechanism of light production in a substance under the influence of radiation is complex and not well understood, there are no theoretical laws to predict the behavior of a given substance in this regard. Briefly, a γ-ray loses its energy in a scintillator through the photoelectric, Compton, or pair-production mechanisms. The electrons thus generated then lose their energy within short distances through ionization and excitation of the scintillator molecules. The ion pairs thus produced then combine among themselves or with other atoms or molecules of the scintillator and produce certain excited states that, during their subsequent decay, emit light. The nature and quantity of these excited states determine the amount, color, and phosphorescent decay time of light.

Properties of Scintillator

A scintillator is primarily characterized by intrinsic efficiency, amount of light produced per unit of absorbed energy (light conversion efficiency), and the time in which emission of light takes place (phosphorescent decay time). The intrinsic efficiency of a scintillator for a γ-ray of a given energy depends on its linear attenuation coefficient, which in turn depends on the atomic number and the density of the material (see Chapter 6). The amount of light produced per unit of absorbed energy, which in effect determines the energy resolution of these detectors, and the phosphorescent decay time, which is an important parameter for the dead time of these detectors, vary from substance to substance.

NaI(Tl) Scintillator

Of all the known scintillators, sodium iodide crystals doped with small amounts of thallium, NaI(Tl), are most widely used in nuclear medicine. Its moderate density (d = 3.67 g/cm^3) and effective atomic number (Z_{eff} = 45) make it very efficient for the detection of x- or γ-rays in the energy range of 30–500 keV. The amount of light produced per unit of absorbed energy in a NaI(Tl) crystal is one of the highest, despite the fact that sodium iodide crystals without thallium doping do not produce much light. The presence of small amounts of thallium (one part in 10^6) enhances the light output by a factor of 10 or more. The phosphorescent decay time, which eventually determines the dead time of a scintillation detector, is ~0.25 μsec and is adequate for the amounts of radioactivities presently used in nuclear medicine. In addition, the technology required to grow these crystals in large sizes and various shapes is well advanced, making their use more economical compared with many other scintillators.

Sodium iodide crystals are hygroscopic and have to be hermetically sealed, usually in thin-walled aluminum or steel containers. Thin aluminum or steel walls attenuate high-energy γ-rays only to a small degree. These crystals should not be subjected to abrupt temperature changes (no more than 10°C/hr change), even when these are not in use (e.g., during shipment or storage). Such changes can produce severe mechanical stresses in the crystal, causing them to crack. Also, the amount of light produced in these crystals is somewhat dependent on ambient temperature. As a result, the response of these detectors changes slightly with change in room temperature.

Light in a scintillator is produced in a very small volume, mainly determined by the range of photoelectrons or Compton recoil electrons produced in the scintillator. For energies of x- or γ-rays less than 1 MeV, this range does not exceed more than a millimeter in a NaI(Tl) crystal. From this small volume of production, light travels in all directions, as shown in Figure 8.5. The direction of most of the light toward the PM tube is achieved by coating the outside surface of the scintillator, except the side facing the PM tube, with a light reflector such as magnesium oxide. The coupling of the crystal assembly to the PM tube is also important because of possible light loss at the interface of the crystal and PM tube. This loss is generally minimized by the use of optical grease.

ASSOCIATED ELECTRONICS
PM Tube

The amount of light produced in NaI(Tl) crystals is quite small relative to that which the human eye can easily detect. Even if one could observe each scintillation occurring in the scintillator with the naked eye, it is not practical to count light flashes in this way. A PM tube is a light-sensitive device that converts light into measurable electronic pulses. It consists of a photocathode facing the window through which light enters, a series of metallic electrodes known as dynodes arranged in a special geometric pattern, and an anode—all enclosed in vacuo in a glass tube. When the light photon hits the photocathode, it produces an electron of low energy (0.1–1 eV) through photoelectric interaction. This photoelectron is then ac-

celerated toward a dynode by the application of a voltage (between 50 and 100 V) to that dynode. As a result of this acceleration, the electron acquires sufficient kinetic energy (50–100 eV) to produce a number of secondary electrons when it collides with the dynode. The number of secondary electrons produced varies between 1 and 10. These secondary electrons are then accelerated toward a second dynode (at two times the voltage applied on the first dynode) where a similar multiplication in the number of electrons occurs. Eventually, at the last dynode (generally the tenth), there are between 10^5 and 10^8 electrons for each of the photoelectrons produced. These electrons generate a current pulse of a few microamperes in amplitude and less than a microsecond in duration at the anode.

The voltage to different dynodes is supplied from a single high-voltage source (500–1500 V) by using a voltage divider. The gain of a PM tube (the multiplication of electrons) strongly depends on the voltage applied to dynodes; therefore, small changes in the high voltage can change the output of these detectors significantly. The crystal and the PM tube are generally combined in a single light-tight unit. This prevents ambient light from reaching the PM tube.

Preamplifier

The electric pulses arriving at the anode of a PM tube are small (microampere) and therefore require amplification to several volts before they can be further analyzed or processed. The output of a PM tube, however, cannot be directly fed into an amplifier because of the wide difference in the output impedance (an important electronic parameter) of a PM tube and the input impedance of an amplifier that results in signal distortion and attenuation. A preamplifier is a device that solves the problem of impedance mismatch. It is located next to the PM tube because long connecting cables at this stage also attenuate the signal. Output of the preamplifier, however, can be sent many feet away from the detector assembly without attenuation.

Linear Amplifier

A linear amplifier amplifies the incoming pulses in a direct proportion. The ratio between the amplitudes of the outgoing and incoming pulses is known as amplifier gain. The amplification can be changed by adjusting the gain control, G, specifically provided for this purpose.

Pulse-Height Analyzer or Single-Channel Analyzer

A pulse-height analyzer (PHA) or single-channel analyzer (SCA) is an electronic device that accepts the pulses whose voltage (height) lies between a preselected range and rejects the pulses whose voltage lies outside this range. An SCA is provided with two controls known as lower level and window that determine the range of the pulses to be selected. For example, if pulses with voltages varying from 1 to 10 are being produced by a linear amplifier in response to an x- or γ-ray, to select pulses whose voltage lies between 5 and 6, it is necessary to set the lower level of SCA at 5 V and the window at 1 V. The SCA will produce an output pulse only when the input pulse lies between this range.

In many instruments, the two controls, lower level and window, have been replaced by peak voltage and percent window. In this terminology, if we wish to select pulses that fall between 5 and 6 V, peak voltage will be set at 5.5 V (center of the range) and percent window = (window width ÷ peak voltage) × 100, which in this case equals (1 V ÷ 5.5 V) × 100 or 18%. Alternatively, a 20% window at 1.40 peak voltage will be 0.2 × 1.40 = 0.28 V wide. In this case, the window is set symmetrically on each side of the peak voltage. Thus, the pulses selected will be in the range from 1.40 − (0.28 ÷ 2) to 1.40 + (0.28 ÷ 2) or 1.26 − 1.54 V. As described later, pulse height can be related to the energy of a γ-ray. As a result, the two controls, peak voltage and percent window, quite often are directly labeled in terms of energy, E, and %ΔE. This, of course, assumes that the volt-to-energy calibration factor does not change with time.

Multichannel Analyzer

A PHA or SCA selects only one range of pulse-height distribution. In a multichannel analyzer, there are many PHAs (1000 or more) that can simultaneously separate the pulses into multiple ranges; therefore, the whole spectrum of pulse-height distribution can be measured at one time.

Scaler and Timer

These devices comprise an electronic counter used for counting the pulses coming from an am-plifier or SCA either for a specific time interval or until a predetermined number of counts has been collected. In either case, both the number of counts and the time during which they are collected are obtained.

Rate Meter

This is a device that instead of giving the number of counts and the time period in which the counts were collected, yields directly the count rate (counts/min). With the ubiquitous use of computers, rate meters are now rarely used in nuclear medicine instruments.

RESPONSE TO MONOCHROMATIC (SINGLE-ENERGY) γ-RAYS
Production of Pulse-Height Distribution

Let us now review the steps leading to the production of the voltage pulse in a scintillation detector. A γ-ray interacts within the crystal through the photoelectric, Compton, or pair-production mechanism. In each case, either a high-energy electron or electron-positron pair is produced that deposits all its energy within a small volume of the site of production. Some energy deposited by the electron or electron-positron pair is converted into light. Light triggers an electric pulse in the PM tube that is then amplified by the linear amplifier.

The height (amplitude or voltage), v, of the pulse coming out of the amplifier is directly proportional to four parameters: amount of energy deposited by a γ-ray (E_d), light conversion efficiency of the scintillator (L_{eff}) that is constant for a given scintillator, PM tube gain (G_{pm}), and amplifier gain (G). In other words,

$$v = \text{constant} \cdot E_d \cdot L_{eff} \cdot G_{pm} \cdot G$$

The variable G_{pm} depends on high voltage applied to the PM tube. If one keeps G_{pm} and G constant, then the pulse height v in a given scintillator detector depends only and linearly on the energy deposited (E_d) by a γ-ray. As E_d increases, so does the pulse height v. The linear relationship between v and E_d, in essence, is the source of the energy-measuring ability of a scintillation detector.

A γ-ray of energy, $E_γ$, however, does not deposit the same amount of energy (E_d) each time it interacts with a crystal. Absorbed energy, E_d, depends on the type of interaction (e.g., photoelectric,

Compton, or pair production). In photoelectric events, all γ-ray energy is deposited in the crystal, that is, $E_d = E_\gamma$. In Compton and pair-production events, E_d is always less than E_γ, and there is no simple relationship that relates E_γ to the pulse height v. Therefore, to perform energy measurement with a scintillation detector, one has to select only the photoelectric events. This is done with the help of a PHA or SCA.

Pulse-Height Spectrum

Figure 8.6 shows pulse-height distribution (spectrum) produced by a NaI(Tl) detector for a monochromatic γ-ray (< 1 MeV) as a result of individual interaction in the crystal of several thousand γ-rays. Here, only photoelectric and Compton interactions are important. The spectrum is divided into two regions, a and b.

Region a is known as the Compton plateau, and pulses in this region originate as a result of Compton interaction. Depending on the amount of energy given to the Compton electron, a pulse of different amplitude is produced. Because in Compton interaction a γ-ray does not transfer all its energy to an electron, the maximum transfer of energy to the electron takes place when the γ-ray is back scattered (see Chapter 6, p. 56). When such an event occurs, it corresponds to the Compton edge indicated by the arrow in Figure 8.6.

Region b, a bell-shaped curve, is known as photopeak. Pulses in this region are primarily produced through photoelectric interaction. A few pulses in this region may also arise as a result of a single or multiple Compton interaction followed by a photoelectric interaction. Thus, total energy of the γ-ray is deposited through multiple interaction rather than a single interaction in the crystal. Multiple interaction from a single γ-ray is much less probable than single photo or Compton interactions. The photopeak is also called total absorption peak.

Because these two regions are generally separated by a valley, the photoelectric events can be easily selected by using a PHA. The lower level and window of a PHA are set to just encompass the photopeak. In Figure 8.6, these may be set at 4.5 and 5.5 V, respectively. A good rule of thumb to select a window width for a γ-ray is for it to be about two times the energy resolution (discussed below) of the detector for the energy of the γ-ray.

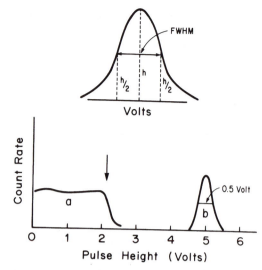

Figure 8.6. Pulse-height distribution produced by a NaI(Tl) scintillation detector in response to γ-rays of single energy. The distribution is divided into two distinct areas, a and b. Area a (Compton plateau) results primarily because of the Compton interaction of γ-rays in the NaI(Tl) crystal. The edge of the Compton plateau (indicated by arrow) results when a γ-ray transfers maximum energy possible in a Compton interaction to an electron. Area b (photopeak) is produced when γ-rays interact in the crystal via photoelectric effect. The narrowness or width of the photopeak is indicative of the energy-resolving capability of a detector. Quantitatively, energy-resolving capability is measured by FWHM. FWHM is depicted in the inset (top) where h is the height of the photopeak.

FWHM and Energy Resolution

Production of light in a crystal and electron multiplication in a PM tube are both statistical processes similar to radioactive decay. As a result, a NaI(Tl) detector does not produce pulses of constant height, v, even for photoelectric interactions where the same amount of energy, E_d, is absorbed each time. Instead, the pulse heights are distributed as a bell shape (Gaussian) in the photopeak. The pulse-height distribution in the photopeak determines the energy-discriminating ability of a detector. The narrower the distribution, the better the energy-discriminating ability of a detector. FWHM is used as a measure of the energy-discriminating ability or energy resolution of a detector. It is expressed as,

$$\text{\% energy resolution} = (\text{FWHM} \times 100) \div (\text{peak voltage})$$

In Figure 8.6, FWHM = 0.5 V and the peak is at 5 V; therefore, % energy resolution = (0.5 × 100) ÷ 5.0 = 10%.

Because the amount of light produced in the crystal for the photopeak increases linearly with γ-ray energy and more light has less statistical variation, energy resolution depends on the energy of a γ-ray. The higher the energy of a γ-ray, the better the energy resolution, although these are not linearly related. Another factor on which energy resolution depends to a slight extent is the size and shape of the sodium iodide crystal. For a well-type crystal, energy resolution is poorer than a cylindrical crystal. Typical energy resolution for a 662-keV γ-ray of ^{137}Cs varies between 8 and 10%. At 140 keV (^{99m}Tc γ-ray), it ranges from 11 to 14%.

Periodic (yearly) measurement of energy resolution is used to diagnose slow deterioration of the crystal due to moisture leaks in the crystal housing and/or the PM tube weakening. Energy resolution gets worse with time as a result of any of these problems.

RESPONSE TO CHANGE IN AMPLIFIER GAIN OR HIGH VOLTAGE

An increase or decrease in high voltage or amplifier gain increases or decreases the pulse-height distribution accordingly, as shown in Figure 8.7. If one has already set the lower level and window of a PHA to encompass the photopeak, then a small change in amplifier gain or high voltage can move the photopeak outside the window. Therefore, it is important that the high voltage and the amplifier gain is stable with time, ambient temperature, and line-voltage fluctuations.

ENERGY CALIBRATION

Because by arbitrarily increasing the high voltage and/or amplifier gain one can produce a pulse of any desired height, v, for a given energy γ-ray, how does one calibrate pulse height to γ-ray energy? This is done by using radionuclidic standard source, which emits a single known energy γ-ray and is long-lived. An example of such a source is ^{137}Cs, which emits a γ-ray of 662 keV.

A calibration universally used in nuclear medicine is that a 100-keV γ-ray produces a photopeak centered at 1.00 V. To achieve this, one adjusts and readjusts the PM tube high voltage in such a manner that the ^{137}Cs photopeak is centered at 6.62 V. Once this calibration has been achieved, neither the amplifier gain nor the high voltage should change. Because high volt-

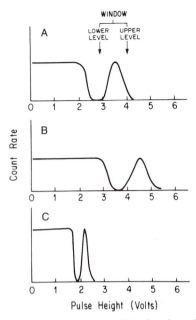

Figure 8.7. Effect of the change in high voltage (or amplifier gain) on pulse-height distribution. An increase in high voltage from that of A produces a pulse-height distribution shown in B, whereas a decrease in high voltage produces a pulse-height distribution shown in C. In these extreme cases (B and C), the photopeak moves out of the selected PHA range completely, thereby reducing the count rate drastically. In practice, small variations in high voltage or amplifier gain can result in appreciable changes in the count rate obtained with a preset PHA setting.

age drifts with time, energy calibration should be checked daily.

RESPONSE TO γ-RAYS OF TWO ENERGIES

In this case, the pulse-height distribution is the sum of the two individual pulse-height distributions of γ1 and γ2, as shown in Figure 8.8. The photopeak of the high-energy γ-ray (γ2) is still isolated, and the low-energy γ-ray (γ1) causes no interference in its detection. However, the photopeak of γ1 lies in the Compton plateau of γ2 and there is no way to avoid the Compton pulses of γ2 from being counted in the PHA window set for the photopeak of γ1. The Compton contribution (leakage) of γ2 in γ1 photopeak, however, can be determined by using a source that emits a γ-ray of single energy very close to that of γ2. With this source, two measurements are made, first at the photopeak setting of γ2 and the second at the photopeak setting of γ1. The second count is the Compton contribution from

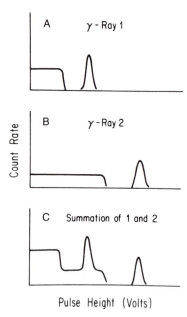

Figure 8.8. Pulse-height distribution produced in response to γ-rays consisting of two distinct energies, 1 and 2. As shown in C, this is an exact sum of the pulse-height distributions produced by γ-rays of energy 1 and energy 2 independently, as shown in A and B, respectively. Low-energy γ-rays do not produce pulses with enough height to cause any interference in the photopeak of the higher energy γ-rays. However, high-energy γ-rays produce pulses with a height corresponding to the photopeak pulses of lower energy γ-rays. Therefore, a correction has to be applied whenever a low-energy γ-ray radionuclide is being counted in the presence of a higher energy γ-ray radionuclide. This is not so in the opposite case.

γ2 at the photopeak of γ1. This is expressed as a percentage of the first count. From this, one is able to correct for Compton leakage in the lower energy peak from the higher energy peak.

SECONDARY PEAKS

Quite often, besides the photopeak and Compton plateau, additional but much smaller peaks can be recognized in a γ-ray spectrum. These should not be confused with the presence of some weaker γ-rays in the radionuclide emissions. Rather, these have well-defined characteristics and causes as described below.

K Escape Peak

This barely visible peak, mostly observed when the energy of a γ-ray lies between 50 and 150 keV, lies about 28 keV below the photopeak of a γ-ray. In this energy range (50–150 keV),

most x-or γ-interactions are through the photoelectric effect in the K shell of iodine atoms and most of these interactions are close to the crystal surface (within a few millimeters). Therefore, the K x-ray produced when the vacancy in the K shell of the iodine atoms is filled has a finite chance of escaping from the crystal without depositing its energy. Thus, in many cases, the energy deposited by the γ-ray, even when the interaction is through photoelectric effect, is not the entire energy of the γ-ray, Eγ, but equals Eγ − $E_{k\,x-ray}$. The energy of the K x-ray for an iodine atom is about 28 keV; hence, the escape peak is 28 keV below the photopeak of a γ-ray.

Summation Peak

With radionuclides emitting multiple-energy γ-rays, sometimes additional peaks corresponding to the sum of individual γ-ray energies are encountered even though no γ-ray with such energy is emitted by the radionuclide. As the name implies, these peaks originate because of the summation of the energies of two different γ-rays in the crystal. Summation of energies occurs only when two γ-rays simultaneously or almost simultaneously (within 0.25 μsec) interact within the crystal. Summation peaks are more pronounced for radionuclides that emit several γ-rays within a microsecond or less of each other and for well-type scintillation detectors (see Chapter 9). Some examples of this type of radionuclide are ^{125}I (28 K x-ray followed by another 28 K x-ray) and ^{111}In (173- and 247-keV γ-rays). If a spectrum is plotted for these radionuclides using a well-type scintillation detector, besides the 28-keV x-ray of ^{125}I, another peak at 28 + 28 = 56 keV is also observed, although ^{125}I does not emit any x- or γ-rays with 56 keV energy. Similarly in ^{111}In, a summation peak at 173 + 247 = 420 keV is observed, although ^{111}In does not emit a γ-ray with this energy. For summation to occur, two γ-rays do not have to interact through the photoelectric effect only. The interaction may occur through the Compton effect as well. Then, the summated pulse, which is also called "pile-up" pulse, will equal the sum of the energies deposited by each γ-ray. At high count rates, pile-up pulses result accidentally, even when the radionuclide emits single-energy γ-rays only.

Back-Scattered Peak and Lead X-ray Peak

These peaks originate from the environment or surroundings of the NaI(Tl) detectors. Because to reduce the background radiation the detectors are generally shielded by lead from all sides except one, the γ-rays interacting with the lead shield produce scattered γ-rays and lead K x-rays of about 80 keV. Some of these secondary radiations can be detected by the crystal. Of the scattered γ-rays from the shield, only those that are scattered more or less in the backward direction have a chance to interact with the crystal. The energy of these back-scattered γ-rays is determined by the expression given on p. 56. The back-scattered γ-rays are not of a single energy but are distributed in a broad range. As a rule, sum of the back-scattered peak energy and the Compton-edge energy in the spectrum of a monochromatic γ-ray equals the photopeak energy.

Semiconductor Detectors

It is not generally possible to measure the amount of ion pairs produced by ionizing radiation in a solid, as is possible in a gas. However, under certain conditions and for a class of substances known as semiconductors, it is possible to measure the amount of such ion pairs produced. The two most common semiconductor detectors use germanium and silicon crystals doped with a small amount of lithium, Ge(Li) and Si(Li). Ge(Li) detectors are used for the detection of x- or γ-rays, whereas Si(Li) detectors are primarily used for the detection of corpuscular radiation.

The principal advantage of a Ge(Li) detector over a scintillation detector is its excellent energy resolution. A typical Ge(Li) detector can easily yield a 1% energy resolution for ^{137}Cs γ-rays compared with 10% using a NaI(Tl) detector.

Figure 8.9. γ-ray spectrum of a ^{60}Co source (two γ-rays with 1173 and 1333 keV energy each) taken with a Ge(Li) semiconductor detector and a NaI(Tl) detector, respectively. With the Ge(Li) detector, the two photopeaks are narrow and clearly resolved. With the NaI(Tl) detector, the two photopeaks are broad and barely resolvable. The energy resolution for a 1333-keV γ-ray is 0.3% for the Ge(Li) detector and 6% for the NaI(Tl) detector. If a third γ-ray with an intermediate energy of about 1250 keV was also present in the ^{60}Co emissions, a NaI(Tl) detector would have been unable to resolve the three γ-rays, whereas a Ge(Li) detector would have identified them clearly.

The main drawbacks of Ge(Li) detectors, severely limiting their application in nuclear medicine, are their low sensitivity, the necessity of maintaining them at a low temperature of 77K (room temperature is about 300K), and their unavailability in larger sizes.

A spectrum produced by a ^{60}Co source and obtained with a Ge(Li) detector is shown in Figure 8.9, where it is also compared with a NaI(Tl) detector.

Key Points

1. Three important properties of a radiation (x- and γ-rays) detector for use in nuclear medicine are its intrinsic efficiency, dead time, and energy resolution.

2. Of these, intrinsic efficiency is the most important. It depends on the linear attenuation coefficient of the detector material and the thickness of the detector.

3. Gas-filled detectors detect ionization produced by radiation in a gas. Ionization chambers, proportional counters, and GM counters are all gas-filled detectors.

4. Ionization chambers are used in dose calibrators because of their stability, although their intrinsic sensitivity is low compared with other radiation detectors. Dose calibrators have to be monitored daily for constancy check and annually for accuracy.

5. GM counters are used in contamination detection and general-purpose radiation-level monitoring. These are portable, inexpensive, and stable devices and should be calibrated annually.

6. Scintillator detectors produce light in response to radiation and are used to detect radiation in conjunction with a photomultiplier tube and associated electronics.

7. Na(Tl) crystal is the most common scintillator used in nuclear medicine. It possesses high intrinsic efficiency and produces a pulse-height spectrum in response to a monochromatic γ-ray.

8. The photopeak voltage is directly proportional to energy of a γ-ray. Energy resolution of a good NaI(Tl) detector is about 10% at 662 keV energy.

9. These should be calibrated daily.

10. Semiconductor detectors have high energy-resolution (1%) but poor intrinsic efficiency.

Questions

1. List the factors on which intrinsic efficiency of a detector depends. Why is this important in nuclear medicine?

2. Is the dead time of a detector related to the maximum detectable count rate directly, inversely, or with some other power?

3. Which gas-filled detector can measure energy of an x- or γ-ray?

4. Why can ionization chambers not be used as a counter?

5. What is the maximum count rate for a typical GM counter?

6. Which detector discussed here is appropriate for the following applications? 1. For surveying the extent of contamination when a technologist, during an injection of a radiopharmaceutical, spilled some radioactive material on the patient's bed and his own clothing. 2. To determine a small amount (0.01 μCi) of radioactivity in a sample. 3. To determine large amounts of radioactivities such as those given to patients. 4. To characterize different radionuclides in a mixture of radionuclides.

7. List the properties of the NaI(Tl) detector that make it so attractive for use in nuclear medicine.

8. What is the function of a pulse-height analyzer?

9. If a PHA is set on the photopeak, what effect will making the window narrower have on the observed count rate?

10. Three NaI(Tl) detectors have FWHMs of 18, 20, and 22 keV for a 140-keV γ-ray. What is the percent energy resolution of these detectors and which one should you select?

In many nuclear medicine procedures, such as the Schilling test, blood volume determinations, protein and fat absorption studies, ferrokinetics, and various radioimmunoassays, it is necessary to determine the amount of radioactivity in a given sample as compared with a standard. In some of these tests (e.g., Schilling test), a radioactive substance is administered to a patient; in others, such as various radioimmunoassays, no radioactive compound is given to the patient. In both cases, however, the choice of the radiation detector and the geometric setup for the measurement of a given radioactive sample is of great importance and is primarily dictated by the overall efficiency (sensitivity) of a particular setup. An increased overall efficiency in these studies allows one either to reduce the radiation dose to a patient or reduce the count time for a given standard deviation error.

This chapter describes the various techniques used for the in vitro detection of the radioactivity of both β-ray and γ-ray emitting radionuclides.

OVERALL EFFICIENCY (E)

The overall efficiency (E) of a given device for the measurement of radioactivity depends on the geometric efficiency of the physical setup (E_g) and the intrinsic efficiency (E_i) of the detector. Thus, the overall efficiency can be expressed as

$$E = E_g \times E_i$$

Intrinsic Efficiency

The intrinsic efficiency (E_i) (see Chapter 8) is defined as

$$E_i =$$

Number of radiations detected by the detector

Number of radiations incident on the sensitive volume of the detector

It depends primarily on the linear attenuation coefficient, μ(linear), of the material of which a detector is made and on the thickness of the detector.

In a scintillation counter, when one restricts oneself to the photopeak counts only, the resulting intrinsic efficiency is known as the photopeak efficiency.

Geometric Efficiency

Geometric efficiency (E_g) can be understood as follows. Let a small sample of radioactive compound be located at a distance from a detector with a cross-sectional radius, r, as shown in Figure 9.1A. Because there is no preferred direction for the emission of radiation from a radionuclide, the radiations (α, β, or γ) from a radioactive sample will be emitted with equal probability in all directions. Therefore, of total number of nuclear radiations emitted in all directions, only a fraction of these will be incident on the sensitive volume of the detector (Fig. 9.1A). Geometric efficiency, E_g, then, is defined as the ratio of the number of radiations incident on the detector from a radioactive sample to the total number of radiations emitted by the sample, or

$$E_g =$$

Number of radiations incident on detector

Number of the total
radiations emitted by source

The geometric efficiency, E_g, for the device shown in Figure 9.1A depends on two factors: the distance, x, between the source and the detector and the radius, r, of the cross-sectional area of the detector. For distances that are sufficiently larger than the radius of the detector (i.e., $x \gg r$), the geometric efficiency varies as $\frac{1}{x^2}$ and r^2, respectively, with the distance x and the radius r. That is, if one increases the distance between the sample and the detector twofold, the geometric efficiency is reduced fourfold (Fig. 9.1B). If the radius of the detector is doubled, the geometric efficiency will be increased fourfold (Fig. 9.1C).

When the sample is very close to the detector (i.e., $x \ll r$), the above relationship ($E_g \alpha \frac{1}{x^2}$) does not hold true. The exact relationship between E_g and the distance x, in this case, is of no practical concern to us here except to know that

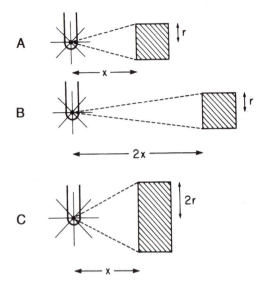

Figure 9.1. Variations in geometric efficiency of a single radiation detector. A radioactive source emits radiations in all directions. Only those radiations that travel in the direction enclosed by the dotted lines reach the detector. The geometric efficiency, which is a measure of the number of γ-rays that reach the detector, depends on the distance, x, between the source and the detector and the radius of the detector as $\frac{1}{x^2}$ and r^2. Thus, the geometric efficiency of arrangement B is one-fourth of arrangement A; the geometric efficiency of arrangement C is four times that of arrangement A. In such an arrangement, however, geometric efficiency can never be higher than 50%.

the maximum obtainable geometric efficiency is achieved when x = 0 (i.e., the source is directly against the face of the detector). In this case, E_g approaches 50%, because even in this situation, one-half of the radiations are emitted away from the detector.

To increase E_g to more than 50%, one either has to use more than one detector or somehow surround the sample from all sides by the detector. The second approach is used in well-type NaI(Tl) scintillation detectors (well counters) and liquid scintillation detectors described below.

WELL-TYPE NaI(Tl) SCINTILLATION DETECTORS (WELL COUNTERS)

In terms of its operation and associated electronics, the well-type NaI(Tl) scintillation detector (well counter) is exactly the same as the NaI(Tl) scintillation detector described in Chapter 8, except that in a well counter, a small cylindrical hole is constructed in the NaI(Tl) crystal to allow a radioactive sample to be positioned very close to the center of the crystal (Fig. 9.2). In this type of detector, only a small fraction (<5%) of the radiations emitted by the sample escapes from the sensitive volume of the crystal; therefore, E_g approaches 95%. The intrinsic efficiency of a NaI(Tl) detector is dependent on the size of the crystal—the larger the crystal, the higher the intrinsic efficiency of a given energy γ-ray. Well counters are available commercially in various sizes. The so-called standard well counter (1.75-inch diameter, 2 inches in height with a hole .75 inches in diameter and 1.5 inches deep) enjoys the most popularity in nuclear medicine. For high-energy γ-rays (>500 keV), however, one achieves a far better count rate with a 3 $\times$ 3-inch well counter than with the standard model. Table 9.1 lists the intrinsic efficiencies of standard and 3 $\times$ 3-inch well counters for various γ-ray energies. It can be seen from columns 2 and 3 that at higher energies, one gains a factor of 1.5 in intrinsic efficiency by using a 3 $\times$ 3-inch rather than a standard well counter. For many procedures, one is interested only in the photopeak counts (i.e., one rejects γ-ray interactions via the Compton effect). In this case, the advantage of 3 $\times$ 3-inch over a standard well counter for higher energy γ-rays becomes even greater (see columns 4 and 5 in Table 9.1).

The overall efficiency of a well counter can be easily calculated. The geometric efficiency for a

Figure 9.2. Geometric efficiency of a well-type detector. Only a small fraction of radiations that are emitted in the direction enclosed by two dotted lines miss the detector. In such an arrangement, geometric efficiency is close to 95%.

small radioactive sample (<1 mL) is approximately 95%; the intrinsic efficiencies for various γ-rays are given in Table 9.1. For a γ-ray with an energy of 140 keV, a standard well counter will have an overall efficiency, E, equal to 0.95 × 0.94 = 0.89 (i.e., 89%); the overall *photopeak* efficiency will be simply 0.95 × 0.88 = 0.84 (84%). One can now also determine the count rate for the photopeak of ^{99m}Tc (140 keV) for a μCi sample. A μCi sample of ^{99m}Tc emits a total of 3.7 × 10^4 × 0.88 γ-rays per second with an energy of 140 keV; 0.88 is the number of 140 keV γ-rays per disintegration of ^{99m}Tc, n_i (see Chapter 2, p. 15). Therefore, the photopeak count rate obtained by a standard well counter will be 3.7 × 10^4 × 0.88 multiplied by the overall photopeak efficiency (84%), or

$$
\begin{aligned}
\text{Photopeak count rate} &= 3.7 \times 10^4 \times 0.88 \times \\
&\qquad 0.84 \text{ counts/sec} \\
&= 2.73 \times 10^4 \text{ counts/sec} \\
&= 1.6 \times 10^6 \text{ counts/min}
\end{aligned}
$$

In these calculations, we ignored the absorption effects of the thin aluminum container of the crystal and the self-absorption in the solution and the absorption by the walls of the test tube containing the sample. In practice, therefore, one will obtain a count rate slightly less than the one calculated above. However, for the present, assuming the overall efficiency as 1.6 × 10^6 counts/min, 10 pCi (10^{-5} μCi) will yield about 16 counts/min. This is a realistic lower limit for the detection of ^{99m}Tc radioactivity by a well de-

tector and clearly demonstrates the high sensitivity of this device. The actual lower limit of detection, however, will depend on the room background and the availability of the time for a given measurement.

The above discussion about overall efficiency pertains only to small sample volumes (<1 mL). How does the overall efficiency vary with the volume of a sample? This can be ascertained from Figure 9.3, where the variation in the overall efficiency of a well counter is shown in relationship to the change in the sample volume (keeping the total activity constant). The addition of 1 mL of dilutant to successive samples progressively reduces the

Figure 9.3. Geometric or total efficiency of a well-type detector as a function of the sample volume (keeping the amount of radioactivity constant).

Table 9.1. Efficiency of a Well Counter

Energy (keV)	Intrinsic Efficiency		Photopeak Efficiency	
	Standard Well	3 × 3-inch Well	Standard	3 × 3-inch Well
80	97[a]	98[a]	97[a]	98[a]
140	94	98	88	96
280	61	80	49	70
320	51	73	36	59
360	48	68	31	50
410	43	66	24	45
510	38	59	17	36
660	32	51	12	25
880	29	46	8	17
1110	28	45	7	16
1170	25	42	6	15
1270	24	40	5	14

[a]Attenuation in sample and sample holder will reduce these numbers slightly.

geometric efficiency. Because the intrinsic efficiency remains constant, the overall efficiency behaves in a fashion similar to the geometric efficiency with the increase in sample volume. The overall efficiency for the same amount of radioactivity in a 4-mL volume as compared with 1-mL volume is about 88% of the latter. Therefore, for a given amount of radioactivity, it is preferable to have the volume of a sample smaller than 2 mL.

The other important parameter of a well counter is the dead time, which limits the maximum amount of radioactivity that can be measured without significant (<5%) count loss. Figure 9.4 shows the relationship of the true count rate to the observed count rate for a typical standard well counter. A good rule of thumb to avoid counting loss due to dead time in a well counter is to keep the total (not just the photopeak) count rate below one million counts per minute. This corresponds to roughly 1 μCi of radioactivity for the common radionuclides, such as ^{131}I or ^{99m}Tc. Hence, any sample containing more than 1 μCi of radioactivity should not be counted inside the well unless one has taken into account the dead time loss. In that case, a simpler alternative to the correction of dead time loss is either to dilute the sample, using a small aliquot of it for counting, or to use another geometric technique such as counting the sample outside the well.

Figure 9.4. Effect of the dead time of the scintillation detector on the count rate.

LIQUID SCINTILLATION DETECTORS

Six elements—hydrogen, carbon, nitrogen, oxygen, phosphorus, and sulfur—make up more than 97% of the total human body weight. There is, therefore, considerable interest in the radioisotopes of these elements both for research and clinical use. The number of radioisotopes of these elements that are easily available and have half-lives long enough for their routine and widespread use is, however, limited to four: ^{3}H, ^{14}C, ^{32}P, and ^{35}S. These radionuclides emit only β-rays (β^-); they emit no x- or γ-rays. The detection of charged particles (β particles, conversion electrons, or α particles) is much more complicated than the detection of x- or γ-rays because charged particles have short ranges in solids and liquids, leading to their absorption in the radioactive sample itself and in the walls or window of the detector before detection. To avoid this problem, it is necessary either to prepare an extremely thin sample and use a detector with a very thin window or to somehow mix the detector and the radioactive source together so that the absorption problem does not arise. This latter alternative is the basis of liquid scintillation counting of β or other charged particles. Liquid scintillation counting, because of its ease and versatility compared with other methods, is the preferred method for β-particle detection, in particular for ^{3}H and ^{14}C, which emit relatively low-energy β particles.

Basic Components

A liquid scintillation detector (Fig. 9.5) consists of two basic parts: a sample detector vial and a photomultiplier (PM) tube and its associated electronics (see also in Figure 8.5, p. 77). Because the latter was discussed in detail in Chapter 8, we restrict ourselves here to a description of the sample detector vial. This vial consists of the radioactive sample and a suitable scintillator dissolved in a common solvent to form a solution as colorless as possible. The scintillator molecules in this solution act as a radiation detector. Homogeneous mixing of the radioactive sample and detector in this manner has two advantages: Because each radio atom of the sample is practically surrounded from all directions by scintillator molecules, the geometric ef-

Figure 9.5. Schematic presentation of a liquid scintillation detector. The electronics used in this case are identical to those used in a NaI(Tl) scintillation detector. However, in a liquid scintillation counter, the radioactive sample and the scintillator are mixed together with the help of a solvent in a sample detector vial (A).

ficiency of such a device is close to 100% and there is little material between the radiation source and the detector (scintillator) to cause the loss of some β particles except for the presence of solvent molecules, which in this case aids in the transfer of energy to the scintillator molecules. Because most effective scintillators are solids, a solvent is essential to achieve a homogeneous mixture of the scintillator and radioactive sample.

The interaction of β particles in the solution with the scintillator, and with solvent molecules, results in the loss of energy, some of which is then converted to light by the scintillator molecules. The amount of light produced in this case, as in a NaI(Tl) scintillator, is directly proportional to the amount of energy lost. Because a β-ray has a short range in liquids and loses all its energy in the solution, the amount of light produced is proportional to the energy of the β-ray. The voltage of the pulse produced by a PM tube in turn is directly related to the amount of light incident on the PM tube. Consequently, the voltage of the pulse produced is directly proportional to the energy of the β-ray. Pulse-height analysis of the pulses produced then allows the simultaneous use of two or more radionuclides with differing β-energy spectra in the same sample (e.g., ^{3}H and ^{14}C).

The sample detector vial and the PM tube are enclosed in a light-tight compartment to exclude the room and other stray light from reaching the PM tube. In modern liquid scintillation counters

the sample detector vial is viewed by two PM tubes rather than one. In this arrangement, using coincidence circuits, electronic noise can be reduced significantly, thus enhancing the sensitivity of low-energy β particles that otherwise will be lost in the electronic noise.

Preparation of the Sample Detector Vial

The main problem in the use of a liquid scintillation detector lies in the proper preparation of the sample detector vial. This requires a careful selection of the scintillator and the solvent.

SELECTION OF SCINTILLATOR

A good scintillator should have a high light-conversion efficiency, sufficiently soluble in the solvent of choice, and chemically stable under a variety of environmental conditions (temperature, humidity, lighting). Among the common scintillators used in liquid scintillation count-ing, 2,5-diphenyloxazole, a p-terphenyl, and 2,5-bis-2(5-t-butylbenzoxazolyl)thiophene enjoy the most popularity. Usually, a small amount of another chemical known as a secondary scintillator is added to the primary scintillator in the solution. The purpose of a secondary scintillator is to absorb light photons emitted by the primary scintillator in the short-wave length regions (ultraviolet and violet) and to re-emit them at longer wave lengths (blue, green, or yellow) that can then be more efficiently detected by a PM tube. The compound 1,4-bis-2(5-phenyloxazolyl)benzene is widely used as a secondary scintillator.

SELECTION OF SOLVENT

The choice of a solvent is dictated by the following requirements: energy deposited in the solvent must be efficiently transferred to the scintillator molecules, the solvent must be transparent to the light produced by the scintillator, and the solvent should be able to dissolve a variety of compounds and be usable at a wide range of temperatures. Toluene, xylene, and dioxane fulfill these requirements and are therefore widely used as solvents. However, because of their hazardous nature, these have been now replaced by safer and better solvents such as di-isopropyl naphthalene. The commercial availability of premixed scintillator and solvent (e.g., Ultima Gold) in a readily usable form has considerably eased the problems in liquid scintillation counting.

Problems Arising in Sample Preparation

The problems connected with liquid scintillation counting do not end with the proper selection of a scintillator and a solvent. The sample, generally a biological tissue, has to be processed in such a way that an almost colorless solution is produced when mixed with the scintillator and solvent. This is achieved either by digesting the tissue in a solubilizing agent such as hyamine (a quaternary amine) or by the more involved technique of combustion and oxidation to produce $^{14}CO_2$, ^3H_2O, and $^{35}SO_2$ that are then easily absorbed or dissolved in a suitable scintillator solvent system. Although the hyamine method has the advantage of relative ease over the combustion and oxidation method, it entails additional problems due to a phenomenon known as "quenching."

QUENCHING

Quenching can be described as any process that interferes with the production or transmission of light from the sample detector vial. This can happen either by chemical quenching or color quenching.

In chemical quenching, the presence of trace amounts of certain chemicals (generally present in the tissue or biological sample) interferes with the transfer of energy from β-rays to the scintillator molecules. Transfer of energy from β-rays to the scintillator is mediated by short-lived chemical species known as radicals. Chemicals causing chemical quenching also react with these radicals but in a nonlight-producing manner, thereby reducing the amount of light produced. In color quenching, the presence of var-

ious colored substances in the sample vial reduces by absorption the amount of light produced, hence lowering the amount of light transmitted to the PM tube.

The end result of this loss of light due to quenching is the diminution in the overall efficiency of the system. This diminution in efficiency varies from one sample to another, depending on the degree of quenching present. For quantitative work, one has to take into account this variation in the overall efficiency. This can be done by counting the various samples first and then recounting them after the addition of a known amount of a standard radioactive substance. The effect of quenching can also be corrected by the use of an external γ-ray source and what is known as the channel ratio method. The details of this method are out of the scope of this book.

PHOTO- AND CHEMILUMINESCENCE

Two other effects that may interfere with the efficiency of liquid scintillation detectors are photoluminescence and chemiluminescence. Because of the property of certain molecules that lets them absorb light and re-emit it at a later time, the sample detector vial continues to emit light for a short time even when it has been placed in a dark room. This phenomenon is called photoluminescence. "Dark adapting" the samples for several hours before counting generally eliminates this problem.

In chemiluminescence, when two chemicals are mixed or involved in a reaction, some light may be produced, depending on the nature of the two chemicals involved. Many biological samples, when mixed with toluene or other solvents, produce chemiluminescence. The only way to avoid the production of light through this effect is to wait for the chemical reaction to be completed (which may take up to several days) before counting.

Key Points

1. In counting, besides the intrinsic efficiency, geometric efficiency is another important consideration.

2. Geometric efficiency depends on distance, x, between the radioactive sample and the detector and area, A, of the detector. It depends as inverse square of x and is directly proportional to A.

3. Well-type detectors have close to 100% geometric efficiency.

4. A well-type NaI(T1) detector has very high overall (geometric × intrinsic) efficiency for x- or γ-rays used in nuclear medicine.

5. Liquid scintillator detectors are the detectors of choice for β-emitting radionuclides, such as ^{3}H, ^{14}C, ^{32}P, and ^{35}S.

6. In a liquid scintillator, the radioactive sample and the scintillator are mixed together in a sample vial. Light produced in the vial is detected with a PM tube and associated electronics.

Questions

1. How can one increase the geometric efficiency of a detector? Does it depend on the type of the detector being used? What are the advantages of 4π geometry?

2. Why do the decay rate of a sample and the observed count rate generally differ? Which one of the two is greater generally?

3. Will the thickness of a sample affect the determination of its radioactivity?

4. Why is the determination of radioactivity of a pure β emitter sample more problematic than a γ emitter?

5. What is the geometric efficiency in a liquid scintillation detector?

10　In Vivo Radiation Detection

Basic Problems, Probes, and Rectilinear Scanners

In vivo detection of radioactivity using external detectors constitutes a major concern of nuclear medicine. This involves a variety of studies that can be divided into two subgroups, organ uptake and organ imaging. In organ uptake studies, we are interested in the uptake of radioactivity by an organ as a whole, either at a given time (static) or as a function of time (dynamic). Some examples of organ uptake studies are radioiodine uptake by the thyroid, renograms, cardiac output measurements, and blood flow determinations. In organ imaging studies, we are not interested in the uptake of radioactivity by an organ as a whole but in the relative distribution of radioactivity in the organ either at a given time (static) or as a function of time (dynamic). For example, in liver imaging, one is interested in the distribution of radiolabeled colloid in various parts of the liver rather than the total uptake of colloid by the liver. Other examples of this group are bone, brain, heart, lung, spleen, kidney, and thyroid imaging.

Although uptake and imaging studies have quite different aims, some problems of in vivo detection are common to both, and the same radiation detector, a NaI(Tl) scintillation detector, is used in both. Therefore, in this chapter, I first discuss the common problems encountered in in vivo detection. I then briefly touch on the specialized instruments (probes) for organ uptake measurement and follow with a brief description of a rectilinear scanner, which is used for organ imaging. Both instruments are rarely used in practice but form an important link in the historical development of nuclear medicine instrumentation.

BASIC PROBLEMS

The use of external detectors for in vivo measurement of radioactivity automatically excludes the use of radionuclides, which do not emit penetrating radiation. Therefore, radionuclides that emit x- or γ-radiation must be used. Three types of problems arise in the in vivo detection of such radionuclides: collimation, scattering, and attenuation. All three factors, coupled with the fact that a detector has to be a certain distance away from a radioactive source (the source being in vivo), reduce the geometric efficiency in in vivo detection by two to three orders of magnitude as compared with the in vitro case (see Chapter 9). This is one of the reasons why millicurie (MBq) amounts are used in in vivo studies as compared with only microcurie or less (KBq) in in vitro studies.

Collimation

Because one is interested in the detection of radioactivity present in a small area or volume (e.g., an organ or part of an organ), it is important to exclude all x- or γ-rays originating outside the area or volume of interest from reaching the radiation detector. This is achieved by the use of a collimator, a device that limits the field of view of a radiation detector. A variety of collimators are available for different purposes. These are usually made of lead, which is inexpensive and possesses both a high density and a high attenuation coefficient for the x- or γ-rays whose energies are of particular interest in nuclear medicine (< 500 keV). A diagram of a simple collimator is shown in Figure 10.1. Note that simple collimation does not allow full discrimination against the radioactivity underlying or overlying the volume of interest. Also, the field of view of such a collimator is determined by two parameters: the length and the radius of the opening (hole) in a collimator. By reducing the radius or increasing the length, one can reduce or narrow the field of view of a collimator to any desired size.

The field of view of a single-hole collimator is related to the spatial resolution and sensitivity of the collimator. Increasing the field of view degrades the spatial resolution and improves the sensitivity and vice versa (see Chapter 12). The field of view also increases with depth; therefore, spatial resolution also gets worse with depth—troublesome feature to be dealt with

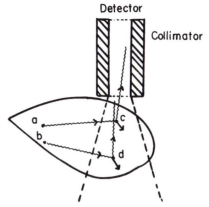

Figure 10.1. A simple collimator. The collimator restricts the field of view of a radiation detector. Only those γ-rays that originate from the radioactive source B can reach the detector, whereas all γ-rays originating from radioactive sources A and C are blocked by the collimator. The field of view of this type of collimator increases with distance from the collimator, as shown by the dotted lines.

Figure 10.2. Compton scattering of γ-rays interferes with the function of a collimator. γ-rays originating outside the field of view from points a and b are able to reach the detector as a result of Compton scattering at points c and d, respectively. The only effective way to reject such events is by the use of pulse-height analysis. The solid arrows at points c and d represent the Compton-scattered electrons. The dotted lines show the field of view of the collimator.

when accurate quantification of radioactivity is desired (i.e., single-photon emission computed tomography [SPECT]; see Chapter 14).

Scattering

The γ- and x-rays emitted by radionuclidic sources embedded in a mass of matter experience, during interaction with that material, scattering via the Compton process. In Compton scattering (see Chapter 6), an interacting γ- or x-ray loses some of its energy and changes its direction. The change in the direction of many γ-rays that originate outside the field of view of the collimator causes them to be scattered toward the radiation detector, thus defeating the purpose of this device (Fig. 10.2).

Depending on the angle of scattering, an x- or γ-ray loses different amounts of energy during Compton scattering. As a result, x- or γ-rays emerging from a monochromatic source embedded in a tissue volume are no longer monochromatic but are polychromatic, as shown in Figure 10.3A. In the case of a 140-keV γ-ray, the energies of scattered γ-rays range from 90 to 140 keV. This assumes that a γ-ray is scattered only once in the tissue. In case of double or triple Compton scattering, which are generally negligible but be-

come more probable as the tissue volume embedding the source increases, the lower limit of scattered γ-ray energy (90 keV) becomes even lower. In diagnostic x-ray imaging, scattered x-rays are reduced by using grids. In nuclear medicine, this can be accomplished by using energy discrimination. Efficiency of scatter rejection with energy discrimination depends on the energy resolution of a detector. When using a NaI(Tl) detector (Fig. 10.3B), pulse-height analyzer (PHA) controls, E and ΔE, are set to accept only those pulses whose height corresponds to the photopeak of the unscattered γ-ray. For an effective job of energy discrimination, the energy resolution of a detector should be very good. For a 140-keV γ-ray, NaI(Tl) scintillation detectors possess moderate energy discrimination capability with full width at half maximum (FWHM) of 15–20 keV as compared with Ge(Li) semiconductor detectors (Fig. 10.3C) with FWHM of 1–2 keV. As a result, a Ge(Li) detector is capable of rejecting almost all scattered radiation, whereas a NaI(Tl) detector does only a partial job. However, despite their better energy discrimination capability, Ge(Li) detectors are seldom used in nuclear medicine, primarily because of their very low sensitivity compared with a NaI(Tl) scintillation detector (see Chapter 8).

The amount of scattered radiation rejected by a NaI(Tl) detector depends on the width of the

Figure 10.3. Scattering of γ-rays in tissues of a patient. (**A**) Monochromatic γ-rays of 140 keV energy from a source embedded in tissue, because of Compton scattering in the tissue, become polychromatic (energy of γ-rays emerging from a patient range from 90 to 139 keV for the scattered radiation and 140 keV for the primary radiation). (**B**) A NaI(Tl) detector, because of its poor energy resolution, detects a significant fraction of scattered radiation in a typical window width used in clinical imaging. Narrowing the window results in loss of sensitivity. Methods 1 and 2 as discussed in text are good solutions to this dilemma. (**C**) A Ge(Li) detector, because of its better energy resolution, detects little scattered radiation in a typical window width used for such detectors but suffers from low intrinsic sensitivity. In **B** and **C**, only photoelectric interactions are shown. Compton interaction in the two detectors from the primary or scattered radiations will produce pulse of less than 90 keV (not shown here) and are rejected by both detectors set on photopeak.

PHA window. The narrower the window, the more scattered radiation is excluded. But narrowing the window to reject scattered radiation exacts a price in terms of reduced sensitivity because more of the primary radiation also is rejected. There are two better ways to reject scattered radiation. One way is the simultaneous use of one more (second) window at a lower energy as shown in Figure 10.3B. The counts or a fraction of counts in the second window are subtracted from the window set at the photopeak. Another way is the simultaneous use of two more windows (second and third) that are only a few keV in width and set just below and above the photopeak as shown in Figure 10.3B. Here, the average of the counts from these two windows is subtracted from the window set at the photopeak. Both methods are better than narrowing the photopeak window because primary

radiation is not lost. However, these methods by no means reject scatter completely and accurately or as much as a Ge(Li) detector does as shown in Figure 10.3C.

Attenuation

Because the depth, shape, and size of an organ containing the radioactive substance are unknown beforehand, the attenuation of x- or γ-rays (absorption through the photoelectric effect and scattering through the Compton effect) in the organ and the tissue overlying or underlying the organ is another serious hurdle in the in vivo determination of radioactivity. As can be seen in Figure 10.4, the distribution of radioactivity varies throughout the cross-section, and x- or γ-rays emitted by a radioactive source, depending on its location, pass through different thicknesses

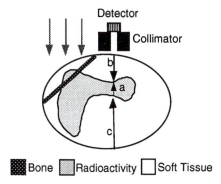

Figure 10.4. Attenuation of radioactivity in in vivo imaging is difficult to correct because the area or volume of radioactive distribution in the field of view of the collimator is unknown (shown by arrow a) and the thickness of the underlying or overlying tissue is unknown (arrows b and c). Point-to-point variations (e.g., at dotted arrows) in these two parameters cause the uniform distribution of radioactivity (per gram or per cubic centimeter of liver) to give different counts at different locations of the detector. Tissues with different attenuation (e.g., bone, soft tissue, or lungs) further complicate the situation.

and often different types of underlying or overlying tissue and therefore are attenuated by different amounts. As a result, a uniform distribution of radioactivity produces different counts at different locations of the organ, not a desirable feature in any imaging.

It is possible to minimize attenuation loss by the use of high-energy x- or γ-rays. The attenuation coefficient for x- or γ-rays in tissue drops sharply with an increase in γ-ray energy up to about 100 keV and levels off with the increase in γ-ray energy above 100 keV. Therefore, radionuclides emitting x- or γ-rays with energies above 100 keV are preferred. Because the sensitivity of NaI(Tl) detectors and the collimators used in scanning decreases with the increase in x- or γ-ray energy, the optimum range of energies for in vivo use is between 100 and 300 keV (see p. 38).

In organ uptake studies such as thyroid uptake of radioiodine, in addition to the use of high-energy γ-rays, attenuation effects are taken care of by measuring a known amount of radioactivity in a standard phantom that reflects the average size, shape, and depth of an organ in a standard man.

In organ imaging studies, generally, attenuation is considered a fait accompli and is taken into account only when interpreting a scan. However, newer imaging instruments fitted with computers can compensate for some attenuation effects by taking images from two opposite sides

and then forming a geometric mean image. Geometric mean, G, of two images or numbers, N_1 and N_2, is defined as $G = \sqrt{N_1 \times N_2}$. Methods of attenuation correction in SPECT are discussed in Chapter 14.

ORGAN UPTAKE PROBES

An uptake probe consists of two basic parts: a NaI(Tl) detector and a collimator.

NaI(Tl) Detector

In in vivo studies, the size of the crystal in a NaI(Tl) detector is an important consideration. Crystal size is determined by the energy of the γ-ray to be detected and the sensitivity requirements of a particular study. For thyroid uptake studies using ^{131}I, the International Atomic Energy Agency recommends that a crystal less than 1 × 1 inches should not be used. A 1.5 × 1-inch crystal is generally adequate for thyroid uptake measurements of ^{131}I and also serves as a multipurpose instrument in the nuclear medicine laboratory.

Collimator

The design of a collimator for uptake studies is dictated by its intended application. However, the following general requirements apply in most cases:

1. To keep the radiation burden to the patient to a minimum, the overall efficiency should be as high as possible;

2. The field of view of the collimator should be well defined but flexible enough to take into account the varying size of a particular organ in different patients while at the same time excluding any radioactivity present in other organs;

3. Because the distribution of radioactivity within the organ and its size, shape, and depth are not known, the overall efficiency or sensitivity should be uniform across the field of view of the collimator and throughout the thickness of the organ.

Because requirements 1 and 3 oppose each other to some extent, one should make the best of a given situation. A typical collimator used in thyroid uptake measurement is shown in Figure 10.5. The overall sensitivity within the field of

Figure 10.5.   A typical NaI(Tl) crystal collimator assembly (probe) used for thyroid uptake of [131]I.

view of such a collimator varies inversely as the square of the distance between the source and the detector but the uniformity across the organ improves as the distance from the detector is increased. For thyroid uptake, a distance of 30 cm is considered optimum.

ORGAN IMAGING DEVICES

Administration of a particular radiopharmaceutical results in its selective localization in the organ or organs of interest in a patient. The distribution of the radiopharmaceutical in an organ may vary within the organ itself, particularly as a result of some focal disease. A diseased or abnormal area in the organ may be hotter (more radioactivity) or colder (less radioactivity) than the adjacent normal tissue. The purpose of organ scanning or imaging is to unravel this relative distribution of the radioactivity present in an organ. Ideally, we should delineate this distribution in all three dimensions (volume), but because of various technical problems, this is not routinely feasible. Instead, a two-dimensional or areal distribution of radioactivity, which is very useful clinically, is obtained. The lack of three-dimensional information in this case is somewhat compensated for by determining the area distribution from multiple directions, generally four: anterior, posterior, right, and left laterals. A two-dimensional record of the distribution of the radioactivity present in an organ is called a scan or an image.

A scanner or imager consists of four elements: a collimator, radiation detector, device to give the location (i.e., x, y coordinates) of the radioactivity, and a system to display the relative distribution in a manner easy to comprehend. Depending on how the x, y coordinates, or information about the location of the radioactivity, are obtained, imaging devices can be grouped

into two classes: rectilinear scanners and scintillation cameras (gamma cameras). Only the rectilinear scanner is discussed here. The scintillation camera is discussed in the next chapter.

Rectilinear Scanner

In a rectilinear scanner, a NaI(Tl) scintillation detector with an appropriate collimator (detector head) is moved over the organ of interest in a straight line with the help of an electric motor. After traversal of a specified distance, the detector head either steps up or steps down a small distance and then continues the straight-line motion in the opposite direction. This back-and-forth motion of the detector head (Fig. 10.6) continues until the area occupied by the organ has been fully scanned. The field of view of the collimator in this case is narrow, and the rectilinear motion of the detector head over the organ generates the span point by point. This type of image formation is similar to that encountered in a television, in which the picture is also constructed point by point, although our eyes do not realize it because of the rapidity of the whole process.

The detector head assembly consists of a collimator, NaI(Tl) crystal, and photomultiplier tube

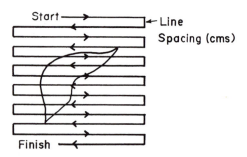

Figure 10.6.   Path taken by the detector head in rectilinear scanning of an organ.

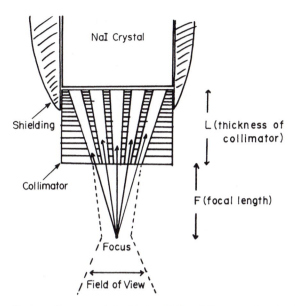

Figure 10.7. Focusing-type collimator. γ-Rays can reach the detector only through the narrow channels as shown by the solid arrows. The field of view of such a collimator (dotted lines) is in general narrow and is narrowest (about 1 cm) in the focal plane. It becomes wider above or below the focal plane.

with preamplifier, all appropriately shielded to reduce room background. Two crystal sizes, 3 × 2- and 5 × 2-inch, are commonly used. The collimator used in a rectilinear scanner is known as a multihole focusing type collimator and is shown in Figure 10.7. It consists of a lead cylinder with a number of tapered holes formed to converge at a single point outside the collimator, known as the focus. The side of the collimator with holes of larger radii faces the NaI(Tl) detector, whereas the side with the holes of smaller radii faces the patient. The distance between the collimator face and the focus is the focal length of the collimator.

The information gathered by the detector head regarding the amount of radioactivity at a given location (number of counts per unit of time) is continuously relayed to a photographic system using a 14 × 17-inch x-ray film, where a small cathode-ray tube, with a fast phosphor screen and well-collimated light spot that exposes the x-ray film, is moved in a light-tight box in synchronization with the detector head. At the completion of the scan, the x-ray film is developed. The count rate (R) observed by the detector head in a given location of an organ is displayed as the darkening of the x-ray film at a corresponding location on the film. Dark areas on the film represent high areas of radioactivity in the organ, whereas light areas on the film denote a low level of radioactivity.

Key Points

1. Three problems, collimation, attenuation, and Compton scattering, make in vivo detection of radiation difficult.

2. Collimation is needed to exclude detection of radiation emitted outside the area of interest. Field of view (FOV) of a collimator is determined by the size of the area of interest. FOV is related to the resolution and sensitivity of a collimator. Collimators are primarily made of lead, an inexpensive, high-atomic-number, and high-density material.

3. Compton scattering in the FOV of a collimator of γ-rays emitted outside the FOV allows some γ-rays to be detected from outside the FOV. The scattered radiation can

be reduced (but not eliminated) with a narrow window set on the primary γ-ray energy in a NaI(Tl) detector.

4. Other methods of reducing the contribution of scattered γ-rays in a clinical situation use two or three windows as described in the text.

5. Attenuation by the overlying tissue is the main source of error in quantification of radioactivity in vivo. In routine imaging, this is taken into consideration while interpreting the images.

6. Organ uptake probes are used to determine radioactivity in a whole organ (e.g., thyroid).

7. Rectilinear scanners were the earliest instruments to determine the radioactive distribution within an organ. However, their inability to detect the radionuclidic distributions at a fast rate made them obsolete.

Questions

1. List the problems that make quantification of in vivo radioactivity difficult.

2. How does pulse-height analysis help in the detection of in vivo radioactivity?

3. What is the primary function of a collimator? Why are collimators made of lead? Can other materials be used instead of lead?

4. Why is there an optimum range of distance between the patient's thyroid and the probe when measuring the radioiodine uptake?

5. Why are rectilinear scanners no longer in clinical use?

Scintillation Camera

A gamma camera, in particular a scintillation camera, occupies a central place in every nuclear medicine department. In a gamma camera, as opposed to a rectilinear scanner where an organ is scanned point by point, the whole organ or a large part of the body is imaged simultaneously. In this respect, a gamma camera behaves similarly to a photographic camera, although the two types of cameras are entirely different in construction and operation. Unlike light rays, x- or γ-rays cannot be reflected or refracted by using mirrors, lenses, or prisms. Therefore, the general principles of light photography cannot be applied to imaging of objects emitting x- or γ-rays. Instead, the selective attenuation and transmission of x- and γ-rays by different materials, such as lead and air, forms the basis of imaging with a gamma camera.

The simultaneous visualization of an entire organ or organs by a gamma camera is its single most important quality that made rectilinear scanners obsolete. This feature makes the study of rapid dynamic processes possible. Dynamic studies with 10–20 images/sec are now routinely obtained to determine cardiac output and ejection fraction.

Of a variety of approaches attempted in research laboratories for the development of gamma cameras, the scintillation camera developed by Anger has emerged as a superior choice in clinical nuclear medicine. Since its commercial introduction in 1966, the modern scintillation camera has gone through several waves of technologic innovations, from improved photomultiplier (PM) tubes and collimators, nonuniformity correction modules, to all digital cameras of the present. It is now almost a new instrument. The only constant element is the scintillator material, which is still a NaI(Tl) crystal.

SCINTILLATION CAMERA

In a scintillation camera, a large disc- or rectangular-shaped NaI(Tl) crystal is viewed from one side by an array of PM tubes. Such an array of PM tubes not only determines the total amount of light produced by a γ-ray interaction, as is common in a scintillator detector and discussed in Chapter 8, but also the location of light production in the crystal. The other side of the crystal is attached to a collimator that acts like a lens of a photo camera.

Physically, a scintillation camera is divided in two parts. The detector head contains the collimator and the NaI(Tl) crystal with PM tubes and associated electronics and is mounted on a stand where it can be easily moved up or down or rotated in any desired position with hand-held controls or automatically under the direction of a computer. Recently, two or even three detector heads have become popular, particularly with single-photon emission computed tomography (SPECT). Increased geometric efficiency is the obvious advantage of multiple detector heads. The second part is the console, which houses the power supplies and operational controls of the scintillation camera, including the display module and quite often an integrated digital computer. In portable scintillation cameras, the detector head and console are joined together in one unit so that it can be moved from one location to another without too much difficulty.

Operationally, a scintillation camera consists of four basic parts (Fig. 11.1, A–D): collimator, detector, multiple PM tubes and position (x, y coordinates) determining circuit, and display. Here, I describe the workings of a scintillation camera. Its operating characteristics such as spatial resolution, sensitivity, and uniformity and quality control are discussed in Chapter 12.

Collimators

The purpose of a collimator in a scintillation camera is to allow x- or γ-rays originating from a selected area of an organ to reach a selected area of the detector. Thus, a collimator establishes a one-to-one correspondence between different locations on the detector and those within the organ. Another feature of a scintillation

DETECTOR HEAD

CONSOLE

Figure 11.1. Schematics of a typical scintillation camera. Four operational components are identified: A (collimator), B (NaI crystal), C (light pipe, PM tubes, and preamplifiers), and D (CRT for display). Detector head incorporates in it A, B, and C, and the console contains D and power supplies and associated electronics.

camera collimator is that its field of view is large enough to encompass completely the total organ or the desired part of the body to be imaged. Four types of collimators have been used with scintillation cameras (Fig. 11.2).

PARALLEL HOLE

It is made of a large number (many thousands) of small holes in a lead disc. The diameter of the lead disc is the same as that of the scintillation crystal used. Thickness of the lead disc and the diameter of the holes depend on the desired spatial resolution and sensitivity of these collimators (discussed in Chapter 12). Lead walls between the holes, called septa, for a well-designed collimator, absorb most, if not all, radiation incident on them. Holes are axial, parallel to each other, and circular or hexagonal in shape.

PINHOLE

It consists of a single hole, about 5 mm in diameter, at the top of a hollow lead cone. The diameter at the base of the lead cone is the size of the NaI(Tl) crystal. The top of the cone faces the

patient. The height of the cone can range from 12 to 20 inches.

CONVERGING

It is similar to a parallel-hole collimator except that the holes, as one moves from the center of the collimator toward the edge of the collimator, start tilting toward the center, as shown in Figure 11.2. Outer most holes have the most tilt. All holes focus at an axial point, outside the collimator (typically 10–20 inches) and toward the radioactive source or the patient.

DIVERGING

In a diverging collimator, the tilt of the holes is away from the center. As a result, these holes converge toward the detector. In fact, if one flips over a converging collimator, it becomes a diverging collimator and vice versa.

As can be seen, in all these collimators, γ-rays originating from one area of the arrow reach only a selected area on the crystal. Thus, γ-rays originating from the front of the arrow reach a different location on the crystal than γ-rays originating from the middle or back of the arrow. The

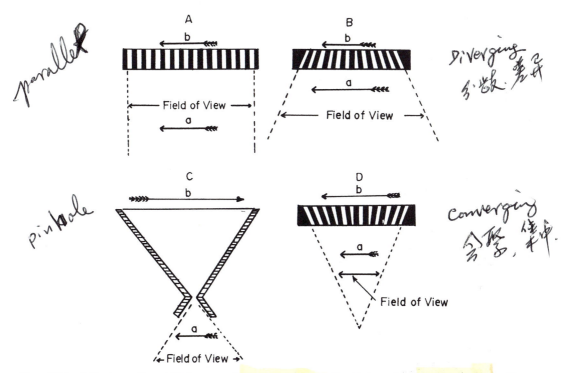

parallel

Diverging
多数.差字

pinhole

converging
分至.佳中.

Figure 11.2. Collimators used in a scintillation camera. (**A**) Parallel-hole collimator: The object, a, projects the same size image, b, on the crystal face. The field of view of such a collimator does not vary significantly with distance from the collimator. (**B**) Diverging collimator: The size of the image, b, is smaller than the size of the object, a, and the field of view increases as one moves away from the collimator. (**C**) Pinhole collimator: A magnified or minified image, b, of an object, a, is produced, depending on its distance from the pinhole. The field of view of a pinhole increases rapidly as one moves away from the pinhole. (**D**) Converging collimator: This collimator produces a magnified image, b, of an object, a. The field of view decreases as one moves away from the detector. A converging collimator provides the optimum sensitivity and spatial resolution for an object that is smaller than the crystal size used in the scintillation camera.

size of the image formed on the crystal depends on the type of collimator and distance of the object (arrow) from the collimator. In the case of a pinhole collimator, the image is also inverted.

The choice of a particular type of collimator is basically dictated by the size of the organ to be imaged. For imaging organs that are similar in size to the size of detector (NaI(Tl) crystal), parallel hole collimators provide the best sensitivity and spatial resolution. For organs larger than the size of the crystal, diverging collimators are preferred. For organs smaller than the size of the crystal, converging collimators have shown great merit. When the size of the organ is small, such as thyroid, a pinhole collimator is the collimator of choice. One problem that makes the use of pinhole, converging, or diverging collimators less satisfactory than parallel-hole collimators is the fact that for three-dimensional objects (which all organs are), the different planes of the object (front, back, or middle of the organ) are magnified or minified to different degrees by these collimators. This produces distortions in the image that under most clinical circumstances are unacceptable.

Commercially, the collimators, besides being characterized by the above four types, are also classified according to their spatial resolution or sensitivity as high-sensitivity (for dynamic studies), all purpose (for most clinical applications), or high-spatial-resolution (for fine details) collimators and according to the energies of γ-rays for which they have been optimized as low-energy (0–200 keV), medium-energy (200–400 keV), and high-energy (400–600 keV) collimators. High-energy collimators are used sometimes with positron-emitting radionuclides, as discussed in Chapter 14. The main difference between collimators designed for different energies is the thickness of septum that increases with energy.

Detector, NaI(Tl) Crystal

SIZE AND THICKNESS

As has already been pointed out, the basic detector element in a scintillation camera is a large disc-shaped [NaI(Tl)] crystal that is viewed from one side by a large number of PM tubes. The diameter of the crystal varies from 11 to 20 inches. Eleven-inch-diameter crystals are used in the standard scintillation camera, whereas 16- to 20-inch-diameter crystals are used in so-called large field of view (LFOV) scintillation cameras. The main advantage of a large crystal is the increased sensitivity for large organs such as lungs or the whole body. For a more effective use of the crystal area, rectangular crystals are also available in some scintillation cameras. The thickness of the crystal is generally $\frac{1}{2}$ inch, but scintillation cameras with $\frac{3}{8}$- or $\frac{1}{4}$-inch-thick crystals are also in vogue, particularly for nuclear cardiology work. Reduced thickness of the crystal improves the intrinsic spatial resolution (to be defined in the next section). The tradeoff for improved intrinsic spatial resolution is the reduction in intrinsic sensitivity, particularly for higher energy (>150 keV) γ-rays.

ENERGY SELECTION

The detection and measurement of energy of the γ-rays passing through the collimator is performed as in any NaI(Tl) detector system except that in scintillation cameras, a large number of PM tubes are used instead of a single PM tube. To determine the energy of a γ-ray, one has to determine the total amount of light produced in the crystal (Chapter 8, p.76). In a scintillation camera, the total light produced is distributed among many or all PM tubes. Therefore, to determine the total amount of light produced, the outputs of all PM tubes have to be summed to produce a pulse equivalent to that produced in a simple NaI(Tl) detector (with only one PM tube). The summated pulse is known as the Z pulse (a misnomer as this should be called E pulse). Pulse-height analysis on Z pulses allows us to select the pulses of the desired energy.

Two important attributes of the Z pulse are linearity with γ-ray energy and its spatial independence (Z pulse-height should not depend on the location of the point of light production in the crystal). On both scores, newer scintillation cameras have improved significantly. The remainder of the nonlinearity and spatial dependence is reduced further by using online correction methods, as discussed in Chapter 12. Summation of pulses from many PM tubes to obtain a Z pulse in a scintillation camera makes its energy resolution slightly worse than a simple NaI(Tl) detector.

Like any other NaI(Tl) detector, in a scintillation camera there are four controls related to the detection of γ-rays and their energies: high voltage, gain of the amplifier, peak energy E, and window width ΔE or %ΔE. Energy selection is usually automated; to choose a γ-ray of a particular energy, one presses a designated button and appropriate pulses are automatically selected. Another useful feature is a provision for simultaneous selection of two or even three γ-rays of different energies. This feature requires two or three pulse-height analyzers (PHAs) and is useful for imaging the distribution of radionuclides that emit more than one γ-ray (e.g., ^{67}Ga, ^{111}In, or even ^{201}Tl) or for rejecting the scattered radiation as was pointed out previously (p. 93).

AUTOMATIC PEAK TRACKING

Scintillation detectors are prone to slow drifts in their outputs, mainly due to the changes in the gain of a PM tube. Changes in the PM gain are caused by small ambient temperature and high-voltage fluctuations. In newer cameras, electronic circuits have been provided that monitor these drifts and readjust the high voltage or amplifier gain to its original value. The automatic peak tracking circuits track the PM gains either on demand or continuously, depending on the manufacturer of a scintillation camera. In either case, the output of PM tubes and therefore the stability of the scintillation camera itself has improved tremendously.

COUNTING

Pulses selected by the PHA, besides being sent to a logic circuit for generation of X and Y pulses as discussed in the next section, are fed into a scaler timer module. The scintillation camera can either count for a fixed-time interval (preselected time) or for an assigned number of counts (preselected counts). There is also a provision for imaging to stop at preselected time intervals or a preselected number of counts, depending on which happens first. A manual control allows one to start or stop counting at any time. Another feature found only in some scintillation cameras is preselection of the information density in a given area of the image. The scintillation camera will stop when a preselected number of counts have been acquired in the desired area of the image. Scintillation cameras interfaced or integrated with digital computers have these functions—start, stop, time, or number of counts—under computer control.

Position Determining Circuit (x, y Coordinates)

PULSE-HEIGHT DISTRIBUTION AMONG PM TUBES

A collimator in a scintillation camera allows γ- or x-rays originating from one small part of an organ to reach a small part of the crystal in a one-to-one correspondence. To keep this correspondence intact electronically, we should know where the γ-rays are interacting in the crystal. This is accomplished with the help of a large number (commonly 37 or 67) of PM tubes, but in Figure 11.3, it is illustrated by considering a simple array of seven PM tubes. In this case, when light is produced at point a in the crystal, it is distributed among all seven PM tubes. However, PM tube 3, being closest to the point a, receives the maximum amount of light. Similarly, when light is produced at other points in the crystal, different PM tubes will receive the maximum amount of light. Thus, by knowing which PM tube received the maximum amount of light, it is possible to know the rough location (near the PM tube receiving the maximum amount of light) of the point of light production. To locate

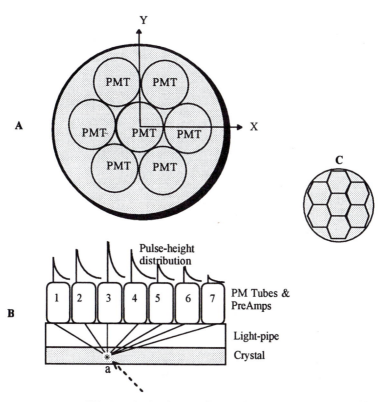

Figure. 11.3.   Geometric arrangement of PM tubes to localize the point of light-production in a scintillation camera (**A**). When a γ-ray interacts at point a in the crystal (**B**), PM tube 3 receives the maximum amount of light, thus providing the appropriate location of the point at which the light is produced. For a γ-ray interaction at a different point, another PM tube will receive most light. By knowing the PM tube that receives the maximum amount, one can approximately locate the point of light production. However, for more accurate localization, we have to consider the pulse-height distribution produced among many PM tubes. (**C**) The shape of PM tubes does not have to be circular; a hexagonal shape is better because of fuller coverage of the crystal area. The same argument is true for the shape of the holes of a collimator where also hexagonal-shaped holes are preferred over circular-shaped holes.

the point of light production more accurately, the amount of light received by each PM tube, rather than the one receiving the most light, has to be taken into account (i.e., the distribution of light among different PM tubes and therefore the pulse-height distribution produced by the PM tubes is considered). The distribution of light or the pulse heights produced among different PM tubes are directly proportional to the solid angle subtended by each PM tube at the point of light production. This fact is used in the determination of the exact location of the point of light production. The PM tubes can be either a circular or hexagonal cross-section. A hexagonal cross-section has the advantage of close packing and therefore less dead space between the PM tubes (Fig. 11.3).

X AND Y PULSES

The output of a PM tube is analog, and it was as such used by Anger to produce two position-determining analog pulses, X and Y. However, in present-day scintillation cameras, the output of each PM tube is digitized (digitization is explained later in this chapter under interfacing with a computer) and all subsequent processing is done with a microcomputer to produce, in digital form, the two position-localizing pulses, X and Y, and the energy pulse Z.

To determine the position-localizing pulses, in analog or digital version, the outputs of various PM tubes are summed with appropriate "weighting factors" (these depend on the distance of the PM tube from the center of the crystal and are not relevant here) to yield four analog signals, known as X^+, X^-, Y^+, and Y^-. In commercial scintillation cameras, the number of PM tubes varies from 19 to 96, and the summation circuits are complex and differ from one manufacturer to another.

The position-defining voltages X and Y and the energy-defining Z pulse discussed earlier are generated from the four voltages X^+, X^-, Y^+, and Y^- as follows:

$$Z = X^+ + X^- + Y^+ + Y^- \tag{1}$$
$$X = K(X^+ - X^-) \div Z \tag{2}$$
$$Y = K(Y^+ - Y^-) \div Z \tag{3}$$

where K is a constant.

The most desirable property of the X and Y pulses is their linearity with distance of the point of light production along the x or y axis from the center of the crystal. The farther the distance (x, y coordinate) of the source of light from the center of the crystal, the higher the pulse heights, X and Y. However, because of the geometry of light collection, these pulses are not as linear with distance as one would like them to be. Use of light pipe as shown in Figure 11.3 or nonlinear pulse shaping are two common methods to improve the linearity of X and Y pulses. These methods do not remove the nonlinearity completely. The residual nonlinearity has to be measured and corrected online, as discussed in Chapter 12.

To display the γ-ray interaction, X and Y pulses (if digital, these have to be converted back into analog form) are used to deflect a light spot on a cathode-ray tube (CRT) or oscilloscope in direct proportion to the amplitude (magnitude) of X and Y. The final image of the distribution is formed from the oscilloscope as discussed under display. If a digital computer is used, this information (X- and Y-pulse amplitudes) is stored in memory for further processing or later display.

INTRINSIC SPATIAL RESOLUTION

Even after considering the amount of light received by all PM tubes and making all the corrections, there is always a small error involved in the exact localization of the point of light production. This error is a measure of the intrinsic spatial resolution of the scintillation camera. Intrinsic spatial resolution is a complex function of the thickness of the crystal, the number of PM tubes used for position determination, the type and shape of PM tubes, and the thickness of light pipe, if used, to couple the PM tubes with the crystal. The most important of these is the thickness of the crystal. Reducing the thickness of the crystal improves the intrinsic spatial resolution, but it also decreases sensitivity of a scintillation camera as a lesser number of γ-rays interacts in the crystal. Therefore, a compromise has to be made between the intrinsic spatial resolution and sensitivity of the scintillation camera. The optimum range of thickness for scintillation cameras is $\frac{3}{8}$ to $\frac{1}{2}$ inches for 140-keV γ-rays. Another factor that also affects intrinsic spatial resolution of the scintillation camera is the energy of γ-rays. This is due to the fact that a higher energy γ-ray produces more light in the crystal (for photoelectric events that are always selected) than a lower energy γ-ray. More light enables better localization of the point of γ-ray interaction, and better localization means better intrinsic spatial resolution. Its exact relationship is shown in the next chapter.

Display

γ-rays originating in the field of view of a collimator interact in the crystal at different locations. These interactions in general occur in a random fashion. A display device should be able to portray such a randomly generated position information (X, Y) quickly (at least 10^6 events per minute) and accurately. A CRT or an oscilloscope, of which a CRT is an integral part, is effectively used for this purpose.

CATHODE-RAY TUBE

A CRT is an evacuated glass tube consisting of five basic components: an electron gun, a focusing electrode, horizontal deflection plates (x direction), vertical deflection plates (y direction), and a phosphor screen. These are shown schematically in Figure 11.4. The electron gun produces a stream of fast electrons. The number of electrons or the intensity of the electron stream can be varied, if desired, by intensity control, I. The focusing electrode allows focusing the electron stream to a narrow circular beam (about 0.1 mm in diameter). When voltage pulses are applied to the horizontal and vertical plates, the electron beam moves in the x and y directions in direct proportion to the magnitude of the voltage pulses applied at the horizontal and vertical plates, respectively. The duration for

which the electron beam stays at its new location depends on the duration of the voltage pulses applied to the horizontal and vertical plates. It is generally less than a microsecond. When there are no voltage pulses applied to the horizontal and vertical plates, the electron beam remains at the center of the phosphor screen. The location of the electron beam on the screen is made visible by the phosphor that emits light at the point where the electron beam strikes it. In this way, when voltage pulses of different magnitudes are applied in succession to the horizontal and vertical plates, the light spot on the CRT screen moves from one place to another but always at a distance that is directly proportional to the magnitude of the applied voltage pulses. The intensity of the light spot is controlled by the intensity control, I.

DISPLAY OF INDIVIDUAL INTERACTIONS

For displaying position information from the scintillation detector, the X and Y voltage pulses are applied to the horizontal and vertical plates of a CRT. The Z signal that carries the energy information exercises a veto on the X and Y signals in such a manner that these are applied to the CRT horizontal and vertical plates only if the Z signal is within the energy range selected by the PHA. If the Z pulses are outside the range selected by PHA, then X and Y are not applied to the CRT horizontal and vertical plates. Thus, only those γ-ray interactions that deposit energy in the crystal in the range selected by PHA are displayed on the CRT screen.

In summary, the display functions as follows.

Figure 11.4. Simplified schematic of a cathode-ray tube (CRT).

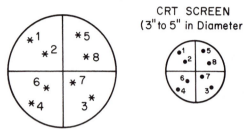

Figure 11.5   Direct correspondence of the location of γ-ray interaction in scintillation detector with the location of light spot on CRT screen.

A γ-ray interacts in the detector and the detector produces three signals, giving the location (X and Y pulses) of the γ-ray interaction and the energy transfer (Z pulse) by the γ-ray interaction. The Z pulse is analyzed, and if it is within the selected range, the position signals (X and Y pulses) are applied to the CRT plates, which deflect the light spot from the center of the screen to a distance proportional to the X and Y voltages. When a new γ-ray interacts in the crystal, a new set of X, Y, and Z signals is produced that then deflects the light spot to a new location given by these signals. In this way, as more and more γ-rays interact in the crystal, the light spot on the CRT screen keeps moving from one place to another in correspondence with the location of γ-ray interaction in the crystal up to 500,000 times or more in a typical image (Fig. 11.5). Because the usual size of CRTs range from 3 to 5 inches in diameter, the image on the CRT screen is displayed in a smaller size than the actual size of the organ or part of the body imaged.

INTEGRATION ON A FILM

A flying light spot on the screen of a CRT does not constitute an image. This image is formed by point-by-point integration of this information on a photographic film.

Film Characteristics

On a film, darker areas represent more radioactivity, whereas lighter areas represent less activity. Film darkening is quantitatively measured by a parameter known as optical density or, simply, density. It is defined as the logarithm (base 10) of the ratio of the intensity of incident light on the film to the intensity of the light transmitted by the film. According to this definition, an area of the film with a density of 2 will transmit only 1% light and will therefore appear almost black to the naked eye. A density of 0 represents 100% transmission; therefore, an area with 0 density will appear white. Densities between 0 and 2 will appear as shades of gray. The relationship of density to exposure for a typical x-ray film is shown in Figure 11.6. This curve is known as the H-D curve of the film. The average slope between points A and B determines the contrast of a film, and the relative log exposure between the points A and B (horizontal distance) determines the latitude of a film. A high-contrast film displays smaller exposure variations than a low-contrast film, but a high-contrast film has smaller latitude. Therefore, the range of exposures that can be displayed on a high-contrast film is smaller (Fig. 11.6).

Film Exposure

It can be seen from the H-D curve that the density is dependent on the exposure or the count rate only in the region that lies between points A and B marked on the curves. The trick in photo display is to correspond this region to the range of the count rates that is of the most interest. Normally, count rates in an organ may vary from zero to a maximum R_{max}. For effective display, R_{max} (also known as the "hot spot") should correspond to point B and zero count rate to point A on the H-D curve. The R_{max} for individual patients differs because of variations in the administered radiopharmaceutical dose, localization and distribution in the organ, and the size and shape of the organ. Some variations are taken care of when one uses fixed number of counts rather than fixed amount of time for exposure. The proper exposure of the film, which is controlled by the intensity I of the CRT, is inversely related to the number of counts. The more counts in an image, the lower setting of I needed and vice versa. Generally, a table is made for the number of counts in an image and I setting needed for proper exposure for those counts.

In fast dynamic studies where the exposure is for a fixed time, the I settings are only a guess. This quite often produces bad results. The only

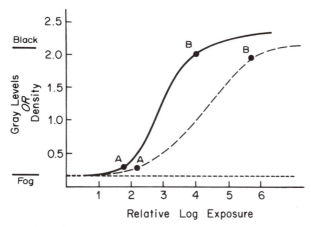

Figure 11.6.   Typical H-D curves of x-ray films used to display information. For the proper display of count rate information, the maximum count rate (hot spot) should correspond to point B and the minimum count rate to point A. Two types of films are shown. Solid curve, film with high contrast and small latitude; broken curve, film with low contrast and large latitude.

solution to this problem is to interface the scintillation camera with a computer, store images, and make exposures after the number of counts in each image has been determined.

Multiformat Recording

A multiformat recording system is commonly used in nuclear medicine. In this system, multiple images are recorded on a single sheet of x-ray film, usually 8 × 10 or 11 × 14 inches in size. The number of images and therefore the size of the image that can be recorded on a single sheet can be varied easily with the help of controls provided for such purposes. Thus, a single sheet may contain from 1 to as many as 64 images. The main advantage of this device is that all views from one patient, including dynamic studies, can be recorded on a single sheet of film, thus consolidating most of the information in one place. A typical study, a bone scan using this format, is shown in Figure 11.7.

IMAGING WITH A SCINTILLATION CAMERA

Generally, the following steps are taken to obtain an image with a scintillation camera:

1. Selection of the study to be performed (e.g., brain, liver, etc.);

2. Selection of the radiopharmaceutical and the dose of radiopharmaceutical. A radio-

pharmaceutical is generally administered to patients away from the scintillation camera, but sometimes, particularly when fast dynamic studies are to be performed, it may have to be administered with the patient in appropriate position under the camera (step 7);

3. Selection of the PHA parameters (peak energy and percent window corresponding to the γ-ray emitted by the radionuclide to be used);

4. Selection of an appropriate collimator (with respect to energy and spatial resolution);

5. Selection of the mode: accumulation of a certain number of counts or exposure for fixed amount of time;

6. Selection of the appropriate intensity of the CRT for the number of counts expected or to be acquired in the image;

7. Positioning of the patient under the camera and, if the radiopharmaceutical has not been administered, administration of the radiopharmaceutical;

8. Start and finish of the exposure;

9. Development of the film. If more than one view is to be displayed on the same film, then the development of the film takes place at the end of the study.

Figure 11.7. Anterior view of a bone scan recorded on a multiformat recording device. In this example, only eight of a possible nine images were recorded.

INTERFACING WITH A COMPUTER OR ALL-DIGITAL CAMERA

Digital computers have acquired an important role in nuclear medicine. The main advantage of a computer is the speed and ease with which it can acquire, analyze, store, and display large amounts of complex data. Presently, scintillation cameras either completely integrated with a digital computer (all-digital cameras) or interfaced with a dedicated digital computer are commercially available. Besides SPECT and heart studies, which cannot be performed without a digital computer, many other applications of computers are now an integral part of standard nuclear medicine procedures (e.g., renogram).

Digitization in General

What does digitization mean? A digital computer handles numbers or digits only and these too in binary (or powers of 2) form only (base 2 instead of base 10). Therefore, any instrument from which data are to be acquired and analyzed by a digital computer in an automatic fashion has to present the data to the computer in binary (or similar) digital form. Unfortunately, most instruments produce signals or data in an analog form. Analog signals are continuously varying and do not produce data in numbers. For example, the needle of a car speedometer moves in a continuous fashion from one end of the dial to the other as the speed of the car is increased from zero to a certain maximum. The higher the speed of the car, the farther the needle moves. The digital (in numbers) information about the car's speed is derived from a scale printed on the dial. The scale printed on the dial is, in a way, manual digitization of an analog (continuous movement of the needle) signal. Now, if the speedometer has to be coupled to a digital computer to record the speed of the car automatically, some electronic device will have to be used that will digitize the information provided by the speedometer (movement of the needle). Such a device, which automatically changes analog signals into digital (binary) signals, is known as an analog-to-digital converter, or simply an ADC. Two important parameters of an ADC, accuracy and speed, are relevant for our purpose. Accuracy of ADC tells how close the numeric data is to the analog signal. Let us consider the example of the speedometer again and assume this time for simplicity that the minimum speed of the car is zero and the maximum speed 100 miles/hr. Now to read any speed in between these two extremes, the scale on the dial has to be divided into equal divisions. If there are only 10 divisions, then we will be able to measure the speed of a car accurately only in steps of 10 miles/hr. When the scale is divided into 100 equal parts, the speed could be read in steps of 1 mile/hr. One thousand equal divisions will provide an accuracy of 0.1 mile/hr and so on. The more divisions there are on the scale (in a given range), the better the accuracy. Similarly, in an ADC, a given range of signals is broken into divisions; the more divisions, the better its accuracy. The unit of divisions in the case of an ADC is a bit. A one-bit (2^1) ADC divides a given range only into two equal parts, a two-bit ($2^2 = 4$) ADC divides it into four equal parts, a three-bit ADC ($2^3 = 8$) into eight equal parts, and so on. The more bits an ADC has, the better its accuracy. However, it takes more time to digitize a signal as the number of bits in an ADC increases. This brings us to the second parameter of an ADC, speed. The faster an ADC is, the higher rates of data it can digitize without any loss of information. Thus, speed and accuracy are inversely related. More accuracy means less speed and more speed means less accuracy.

Digitization in the Scintillation Camera

In a scintillation camera, unless it is an all-digital scintillation camera, in which case the digitization has already been done at the PM tube, the X, Y, and Z pulses are analog and have to be digitized before being recorded by a digital computer. The ADCs used for digitizing X and Y signals of a scintillation camera are 7–9 bits, which means that the X and Y ranges are equally divided into $2^7 = 128$, $2^8 = 256$, or $2^9 = 512$ equal divisions, respectively. In a scintillation camera, the maximum range of X or Y signals will equal the diameter of the crystal. Therefore, each division of an ADC will correspond to either d/128 or d/256 cm of distance, depending whether the ADC is 7 or 8 bit. For an 11-inch- (28 cm) diameter crystal and 7-bit ADC or for an LFOV (20-inch-diameter) crystal and 8-bit ADC, this value equals 0.2 cm. Because the intrinsic spatial resolution of a scintillation camera presently is in this range, greater accuracy is not needed. In terms of the speed of the ADC, it should be able to handle about 100,000 signals per second, because higher count rates are seldom encountered in nuclear medicine.

The digitization of X and Y signals into 64, 128, or 256 divisions yields a 64 × 64, 128 × 128, or 256 × 256 matrix. Thus, the analog image (which is two dimensional or areal distribution) is divided into 64 × 64 = 4096, 128 × 128 = 16384, or 256 × 256 = 65536 equal small areas known as pixels. A specific area on the crystal corresponds to a specific pixel, and each pixel is assigned a specific location in the computer memory. Therefore, when a γ-ray interacts in the crystal, its pixel location is determined by the ADCs and a count is stored in the corresponding location in the computer. As more and more γ-rays interact, they are stored in the appropriate locations, and finally a digitized image is formed. This is graphically illustrated in Figure 11.8 using a 4 × 4 matrix instead of 64 × 64, 128 × 128, or 256 × 256, which are used in practice.

SOME APPLICATIONS OF COMPUTERS

The various areas where the computer has helped tremendously in the practice of nuclear medicine are as follows.

Figure 11.8.   Digitization of an image. Analog image produced by a scintillation camera is divided into a number of (4000 or 16,000) square cells or pixels. Counts from each pixel are stored in a separate location in a computer. Here, the X,Y ranges have been divided into four divisions. The resultant 4 × 4 matrix has 16 pixels.

Automatic Acquisition of Images

In the case of static imaging, a digital computer is not as helpful as in the case of fast dynamic studies where images may have to be acquired every 0.5 second for a period of 100 seconds or more. In dynamic studies, a digital computer is the only practical way to acquire such a large amount of data accurately and efficiently. Another type of acquisition, known as multiple gated acquisition (MUGA), is also made practical by computer acquisition of data. MUGA is desired where the organ to be imaged moves in a periodic fashion (e.g., heart) (Fig.

11.9). To acquire images in various phases of a heart beat (such as systole or diastole), the beat is divided into a number of time segments, usually 16. Each time segment corresponds to a particular phase of the heart beat. Onset of the first time segment is triggered by the R wave of an electrocardiogram monitor attached to the patient, and data during this segment is collected in a designated area of the computer memory, called frame 1. At the end of this time segment, data acquisition for the second time segment takes place in a different location of the computer memory, called frame 2. Thus, data recorded by the scintillation camera during each

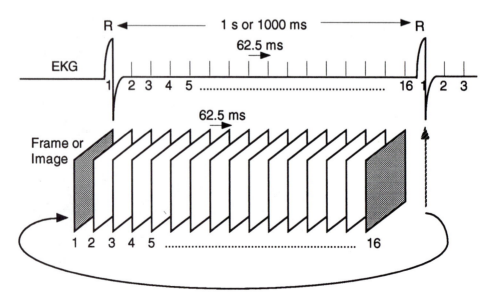

Figure 11.9.   Schematic representation of a heart beat and its division into time segments and the corresponding frames or images of computer memory for heart studies in a multiple gated acquisition (MUGA).

time segment (62.5 msec in this example) are stored by computer in different parts of its memory, called frames or images (16 in this case). Each time segment corresponds to a particular frame or image. When the next beat starts, as indicated by the second R wave, the data acquisition reverts back into frame 1 for the first time segment and frame 2 for the second time segment and so on. This process continues for a large number of beats, quite often up to 1000 or more. The reason for summing the data for each time segment of a heart beat for so many heart beats has to do with the number of counts in the image of each time segment (also called "gate").

Because a heart beat is generally less than one second in duration, if one divides it into 16 time segments, each time segment is only 30–70 msec (depending on the actual time of the beat). The number of counts detected by the scintillation camera during a 30- to 70-msec time interval, even for a 20-mCi ^{99m}Tc dosage to the patient, is quite small. Therefore, by adding counts from a large number of beats for each time segment, images with sufficient numbers of counts (200,000–1,000,000) for each time segment of heart cycle (phase) can be obtained. Images thus obtained from one patient are shown in Figure 11.10.

Display of Images

In scintillation camera imaging, even with a multi-imager, the proper intensity setting of the oscilloscope light spot in every case is difficult. With computer-acquired digital images,

Figure 11.10.   Sixteen images in different phases of heart beat acquired with MUGA.

there is no such problem. Images can be stored temporarily or permanently on a disc or magnetic tape and displayed over and over again with any desired intensity level (Fig. 11.11). The dynamic images can be displayed in a movie-like fashion so that the flow of a bolus of radioactivity can be followed. MUGA images of the heart (Fig. 11.10) can be displayed in a ciné mode, which shows the motion of the heart during a heart beat. Obviously, this cannot be illustrated here.

Analysis of the Images

The digitized images can be manipulated individually or added, subtracted, multiplied, or divided by one another by the computer to generate another image, which may provide better appreciation of certain clinically important parameters. Also, counts can be determined and compared from areas of interest in the same images or in images taken at different times. An example is the heart study of Figure 11.10. By drawing regions of interest for the left ventricle in each of the 16 frames, one obtains the left ventricle volume in each phase of the heart, and it can be represented as a function of time. From the two phases at diastole and systole, one computes the ejection fraction of the heart. This is shown in Figure 11.12. Another example of the use of the digital computer in a dynamic study in the brain is depicted in Figure 11.13.

Figure 11.11. Same lung study shown with four different display intensities. Optimum intensity setting is important for accurate diagnosis.

Figure 11.12.   (**A**) Regions of interest (ROI) in systole and distole and (**B**) left ventricle volume as a function of time during one heart beat.

Figure. 11.13. Use of a computer to acquire, analyze, and display nuclear medicine images. Sequential brain images of 1-second duration were acquired for 50 seconds. From these data, a composite image consisting of all 50 1-second images was formed (**A**). The areas of interest (left and right hemisphere) were chosen. The computer then formed dynamic curves showing time changes in the two regions of interest (**B**). Also shown (**C**) are the first 16 2-second images formed by adding 2 1-second images successively.

Key Points

1. A scintillation camera can image radionuclidic distributions at a fast rate (20 images/sec). It is available with single, dual, and triple heads and in various crystal sizes.

2. It consists of four operational components, a collimator, a NaI(Tl) crystal, a large number of PM tubes and associated electronics to determine the location of γ-ray interaction in the crystal, and a display system consisting of an oscilloscope and a photographic camera.

3. Four types of collimators, parallel hole, converging, diverging, and pinhole, have been used. Parallel-hole collimator is the optimum collimator for most studies performed in nuclear medicine.

4. The size of the crystal depends on the use of the scintillation camera. For cardiac studies only, small fields of view (10 inch diameter) scintillation cameras are sufficient, but for the whole body studies, LFOV scintillation cameras are needed. The thickness of the crystal is normally 0.5 inches but slightly less for a dedicated cardiac unit.

5. Thickness of the crystal is inversely related to the intrinsic spatial resolution of the scintillation camera.

6. Output of the PM tubes is combined in a weighted manner to generate three signals: X, Y, and Z. The two position signals, X and Y, are proportional to the x and y distance of the point of γ-ray interaction in the crystal from the center of the crystal. The Z signal at the photopeak is proportional to the energy of the γ-ray.

7. The position signals, X and Y, deflect a light spot proportional to the distance from the center of the point of interaction in the crystal on an oscilloscope from where the image is obtained with camera.

8. Newer scintillation cameras are all digital and have a computer as an integral part. Analog scintillation cameras can be easily interfaced with a computer.

9. A computer allows an automated acquisition, different gray-scale displays, and quantification and processing of images.

Questions

1. The crystal in a scintillation camera has an optimum thickness. What are the two properties that determine the optimum thickness?

2. If, in the future, a new scintillator material is discovered that produces four times the amount of light produced by the NaI(Tl) crystal for a 140-keV γ-ray, what factor of the scintillation camera can be affected and how?

3. Name the collimator for which each of the following statements is true: (a) The field of view remains constant. (b) It magnifies the object. (c) Its field of view increases with distance and it minifies the object. (d) It inverts the object.

4. For optimum exposure of the film, how should the intensity of the light spot of the oscilloscope be changed if the number of counts in the image is increased?

5. An ADC is the most important link between a scintillation camera and a digital computer. If the spatial resolution of the scintillator camera improves by a factor of 10, what effect will it have on the desired accuracy and speed of the ADC?

12 Operational Characteristics and Quality Control of a Scintillation Camera

A number of parameters of an imaging device play a major role in the delineation of a radioactive distribution. Of these, two, spatial resolution and sensitivity, are important. For scintillation cameras, two other operational characteristics, uniformity and high count rate performance, are also considered. These and some routine quality control procedures constitute the subject matter of this chapter.

QUANTITATIVE PARAMETERS FOR MEASURING SPATIAL RESOLUTION

Spatial resolution is defined as the ability of an imager to reproduce the details of radionuclidic distribution. The finer the details an imaging device reproduces, the better spatial resolution it has. How is spatial resolution measured quantitatively? Two parameters—full width at half maximum (FWHM) of a point-spread function and modulation transfer function (MTF)—are used to measure spatial resolution of an imaging device. Sometimes "bar phantoms" are used as a semiquantitative measure of spatial resolution. These are discussed later in this chapter (p.123).

Point-Spread Function and FWHM

If we image a single point source and plot the intensity profile across its center, a bell-shaped curve similar to that shown in Figure 12.1 results. This curve is known as the point-spread function of an imager. The FWHM of this curve can be used to measure spatial resolution quantitatively. The unit of resolution is the same as the unit of length, centimeter, or millimeter generally. A narrower FWHM implies a better spatial resolution of the imaging device. Thus, an imaging device with 2 mm FWHM is a better imaging device than one with 5 mm FWHM. Measurement of FWHM is quite involved and requires a computer interfacing with a scintillation camera.

FWHM is a useful parameter for expressing the relationship of spatial resolution to various parameters of an imaging device such as size, shape, and length of the holes of a collimator of a scintillation camera. Its main drawback is that it does not measure spatial resolution under varying object contrast conditions. As a result, it is possible to design two imaging devices that have equal spatial resolutions according to this definition, although in practice one performs better than the other.

Modulation Transfer Function

MTF gives the most complete characterization of the spatial resolution of an imaging device, provided that the response of the imaging device is linear. Although the latter condition is not strictly met for imaging devices, the MTF is still useful in their evaluation. Its main drawback is the inability to express its relationships with the various parameters of an imaging device in simple and understandable terms.

To understand this parameter fully, knowledge of Fourier analysis is essential. However, to comprehend it conceptually, an analogy with sound is helpful. Any sound—the ding-dong of a bell or the pretty voice of a singer—is made up of a number of sound waves of different frequencies. Once the component frequencies and their strengths (amplitudes) are known for a given sound, it can then be resynthesized (in a laboratory) by proper superimposition of these frequencies. In a similar fashion, any spatial distribution (object) can be broken down into a number of spatial frequencies, and the original distribution (object) can then be resynthesized by the proper superimposition of these spatial frequencies.

How does this breaking up of a spatial distribution into component spatial frequencies aid in evaluating the imaging device? Not per se, but if we measure the degradation produced by an imaging device as a function of various spatial frequencies, the resulting function will provide the information needed to characterize the imaging system completely. The degradation (M) pro-

Figure 12.1. Intensity profile through the center of a point source image with a scintillation camera. The width or narrowness of such a profile is a good measure of spatial resolution. The narrower the curve, the better the spatial resolution of the imager. The full width of this curve at the two points for which the response has decreased to one half of the maximum (FWHM) is customarily used as a quantitative parameter for measuring the spatial resolution of an imaging device.

duced for a spatial frequency v by an imaging device is measured as the ratio of the contrast (amplitude of the wave) in the image frequency to the contrast in the object frequency (Fig. 12.2).

Measurement of M as a function of v, then, produces the MTF of the imaging device. When the value of M for a particular spatial frequency is 1, this indicates no degradation of contrast for that frequency. If M equals zero, the imaging device is unable to reproduce this particular spatial frequency; therefore, a value of zero represents the maximum degradation. Values of M between 1 and 0 represent the extent of degradation for a given frequency. An ideal imager (which produces an exact image of an object) will have a value of M = 1 for all spatial frequencies.

Use of the MTF to compare the spatial resolution of two different imaging devices can be appreciated easily by examining Figure 12.3, which depicts the MTF for three imaging devices, A, B, and C, respectively. Here, the MTF of the imaging device A is higher for all spatial frequencies than the MTF of the imaging devices B and C; therefore, the imaging device A possesses the best spatial resolution of the three imaging devices. The choice between B and C is difficult. At low spatial frequencies, B is superior to C, whereas at higher frequencies C is superior to B. The selection of the particular imaging device in this case will depend on the type of objects to be imaged. If an object dominates in high frequencies, device C will be a better choice. If an object contains primarily low frequencies, then device B will be more advantageous to use. The MTF of an imaging device is difficult to measure directly. Instead, it is calculated from the line-spread function (discussed below) of an imager, which can be easily measured.

Resolution of an Imaging Chain

Quite often an imaging device can be broken into components, with each component contributing to the final or system resolution of the imaging device; for example, in the case of scintillation camera, the final or system resolution is derived from two components, the collimator and the x,y localization mechanism. How does one combine these component resolutions to give the system resolution. If the resolution is expressed using FWHM and $R_1, R_2 \ldots$ are the

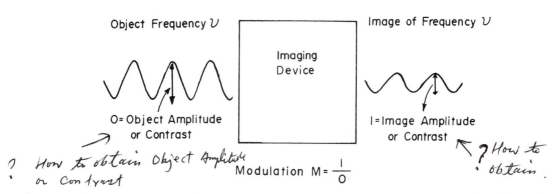

Figure 12.2. Modulation transfer function (MTF). When a spatial frequency, v, of an object is imaged, its amplitude may change. The ratio of the amplitude in the image of a spatial frequency to that in the object is known as modulation, M. Measurement of M as a function of v yields the MTF of an imaging device.

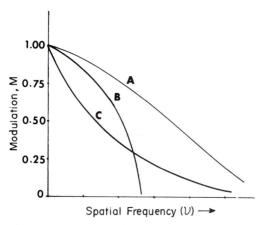

Figure 12.3. MTF of three imaging devices. Modulation M for imaging device A is higher than that of B and C at all spatial frequencies. Therefore, it possesses the best spatial resolution of the three. The choice between B and C is difficult because at low spatial frequencies, B is superior to C, whereas at high spatial frequencies, C is superior to B.

component resolutions, respectively, then the system resolution R_s, is given as follows:

$$R_s = \sqrt{R_1^2 + R_2^2 + \ldots} \qquad [1]$$

For MTF representation of resolution, the system, MTF_s, is given by the following expression:

$$MTF_s = MTF_1 \cdot MTF_2 \cdot \ldots \qquad [2]$$

QUANTITATIVE PARAMETERS FOR MEASURING SENSITIVITY

In addition to spatial resolution, the other important parameter of an imaging device is sensitivity. Sensitivity can be defined as the ability of an imaging device to use efficiently all the photons available from an object within a given unit of time. Three parameters—point sensitivity, line sensitivity, and plane sensitivity—have been used to measure the sensitivity of an imaging device. Each has relative advantages and disadvantages.

Point Sensitivity (S_p)

This parameter is defined as the fraction of γ-rays detected per unit of time for a point source of radioactivity. In a scintillation camera, S_p is more or less constant in the field of view of the collimator.

Line Sensitivity (S_L)

This parameter is defined as the fraction of γ-rays detected per unit of time per unit of length

of a very long line source of uniform radioactivity. The count profile of a line source, as determined by an imaging device, through a direction perpendicular to the line source is known as the line-spread function (LSF) (Fig. 12.4). LSF(x) is primarily used in the calculation of the MTF of an imager as follows:

$$MTF(\nu) = \frac{\int_{-\infty}^{\infty} LSF(x) \cdot \cos(2\pi\nu x) \cdot dx}{\int_{-\infty}^{\infty} LSF(x) \cdot dx} \qquad [3]$$

Plane Sensitivity (S_A)

Plane sensitivity is defined as the fraction of γ-rays detected per unit of time per unit of area of a large plane source of uniform radioactivity. This parameter is commonly used to compare the sensitivities of two imaging devices. The principal advantage of S_A is the ease with which it can be measured. Plane sensitivity does not vary with the distance of the plane source from the collimator as long as the area of the plane source is larger than the field of view of the collimator at that distance.

FACTORS AFFECTING SPATIAL RESOLUTION AND SENSITIVITY OF AN IMAGER

The spatial resolution and sensitivity of an imaging device depend on a number of variables described below. Theoretically, the exact relationships of these variables to spatial resolution and sensitivity are difficult to obtain in a generalized case. However, by making certain assumptions, these relationships can be expressed in simplified mathematical form. Using these formulas, an approximation of the dependence of spatial resolution and sensitivity on a given

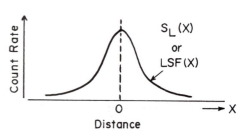

Figure 12.4. LSF of an imaging device. Using a gamma camera, LSF can be directly obtained from the image of a line source, provided it is interfaced with a computer system.

variable can be easily deduced. In the following discussion, we use these simpler formulas. In addition, we use R (FWHM) and S_A as a measure of the spatial resolution and sensitivity, respectively, of an imaging device, assuming that there is no septal penetration by γ-rays in the collimator of the scanner and there is no scattering of γ-rays in the radionuclide source.

Scintillation Camera

The spatial resolution, R_s, of a scintillation camera is comprised of R_1 and R_2, where R_1 is the intrinsic spatial resolution of a scintillation camera and R_2 is the spatial resolution of the collimator used with the scintillation camera. Spatial resolution, R_s, is approximately related to R_1 and R_2 as by equation (1).

The intrinsic spatial resolution R_1, which is a measure of the uncertainty in the localization of the point where light is produced in the crystal, is degraded with an increase in the thickness of the NaI(Tl) crystal and is improved with an increase in γ-ray energy. The improvement in the intrinsic spatial resolution of a camera with the γ-ray energy is shown in Figure 12.5.

Spatial resolution R_2 depends on various collimator parameters such as collimator length, L, and diameter of holes, d. We limit our discussion here to a parallel-hole collimator (Fig. 12.6), although similar considerations apply for a converging or diverging collimator. R_2 in this case depends on the hole diameter d, length of

$$R_2 \simeq \frac{d(L+F+c)}{L}$$

Figure 12.6. Dependence of spatial resolution, R_2, of a parallel-hole collimator on the length, L, of the collimator and the diameter, d, of the holes. Reducing d or increasing L improves R_2. Sensitivity of such a collimator also varies as inverse square of the spatial resolution.

the collimator L, thickness of the crystal c, and the distance F of the source from the collimator face. R_2 is given by the following expression:

$$R_2 \cong \frac{d(L + F + c)}{L} \qquad [4]$$

When the source is at a distance F from the collimator, to improve R_2, we have to either reduce d and c or increase L.

The sensitivity S_A depends on d, L, D (crystal diameter), ε_p (intrinsic efficiency), and s (septa thickness), as follows:

$$S_A \cong \frac{\pi d^4}{64L^2} \cdot \frac{3D^2}{4(d + s)^2} \cdot \varepsilon_p \qquad [5]$$

It can be seen from equation (5) that S_A can be increased by either increasing d or decreasing L, the opposite of that required to improve the spatial resolution R_2 (for an optimum collimator, $S_A \propto R_2^2$). Therefore, a twofold improvement in R_2 (keep in mind that improvement in resolution means that R_2 has to decrease in value), either by decreasing d or by increasing L, necessitates a fourfold sacrifice in S_A. Sensitivity of a parallel-hole collimator can be increased by enlarging the diameter D of the crystal ($S_A \propto D^2$). Accordingly, a 13-inch-diameter crystal scintillation camera has a sensitivity equal to ($13^2/11^2$), or 1.4 times that of an 11-inch-diameter crystal scintillation camera. This gain in sensitivity of a large crystal scintillation camera is of value only in cases

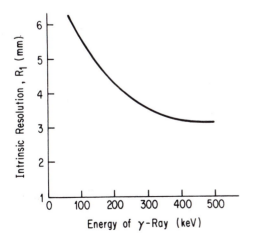

Figure 12.5. Dependence of intrinsic spatial resolution (R_1) of an Anger camera on γ-ray energy.

where the organs to be imaged are of the same size as the crystal. Sensitivity can also be increased by improving ε_p by making the crystal thicker, particularly for higher energy γ-rays. Of course, that will degrade the intrinsic resolution.

Loss of Spatial Resolution Resulting From Septal Penetration

In the previous discussion, we assumed that no γ-ray could reach the radiation detector by penetrating the septa of the collimator. Such an assumption is justifiable only in the case of collimators designed for use with low-energy γ-rays (<150 keV). In collimators designed for use with high-energy γ-rays, some septal penetration always occurs because a further reduction of septal penetration, by increasing septal thickness, will produce an unacceptable loss in the sensitivity of the collimator.

The effect of septal penetration on the spatial resolution of a collimator is to degrade it. Septal penetration, in effect, may be construed as an effective increase in the diameter, d, of the collimator holes. The extent of the degradation of spatial resolution depends on the degree of septal penetration. Higher penetration leads to greater degradation of spatial resolution.

Variation in Spatial Resolution With Depth

Spatial resolution of a scintillation camera varies with the depth or distance from the face of the collimator. For the scintillation camera, the best spatial resolution is achieved at the face of the collimator. The farther away from the face of the collimator, the poorer the spatial resolution. The dependence of spatial resolution on depth of a typical parallel-hole collimator of a scintillation camera is shown in Figure 12.7, where both R and MTF were used as the index of spatial resolution.

UNIFORMITY AND HIGH COUNT RATE PERFORMANCE OF A SCINTILLATION CAMERA

Besides spatial resolution and sensitivity, two other characteristics of a scintillation camera, uniformity and high count rate performance, are also important for the optimal operation of a scintillation camera.

Figure 12.7. Variation of the spatial resolution of a scintillation camera with depth. The best spatial resolution is obtained closest to the collimator. In **A,** R has been used as a measure of spatial resolution; in **B,** MTF has been used for this purpose. Both, however, show similar behavior in variation of spatial resolution with depth. The number on the MTF curves in **B** gives the distance from the collimator face.

Uniformity

It is the ability of a scintillation camera to reproduce a uniform radioactive distribution (mind you, in a uniform source, there are no details or variations of count rate; therefore, spatial resolution has little to do with the uniformity response of a scintillation camera). In practice, all scintillation cameras produce nonuniform or inhomogeneous images of a uniform source to varying extent. These inhomogeneities or the count rate variations from one area to another in the image of a uniform source may be in amounts up to ±10%. In the uncorrected image, these areas show as increased ("hot") or decreased ("cold") spots of radioactivity as depicted in Figure 12.8), taken from an old scintillation camera.

Although some inhomogeneity in the image of a uniform source is caused by slight variations in the thickness of the NaI(Tl) crystal and in the transmission of the γ-rays by the collimator, the dominant cause of nonuniform response is electronic in nature. It is related to differences in response of photomultiplier (PM) tubes and to the difference in transmission of light produced at

Figure 12.8. Uncorrected "flood" showing the nonuniform response of an old scintillation camera with a hexagonal crystal. The bright outer ring in the image is due to edge packing. In new cameras, this ring is no longer visible.

different places in the crystal. These differences cause the mispositioning of some counts. A good demonstration of mispositioning of counts occurs in scintillation cameras occasionally when a straight-line radioactive source is imaged. The image of a linear radioactive source appears as an arc, which may be curved in or out from the center of the scintillation camera (pin cushion or barrel distortion in optical analogy). Such distortions of linear sources are visible only when the scintillation camera is not properly "tuned." A certain amount of nonlinearity always persists even when it is not discernible on visual inspection of the image and the camera is properly tuned. These small nonlinearities result in a visible nonhomogeneous response of the scintillation camera to a uniform source. To keep the nonhomogeneities to a minimum, scintillation cameras must be properly tuned. Tuning involves the readjustment of individual PM tube gains so as to overcome the individual differences in various PM tube responses. Because the PM tube gain may drift as a result of fluctuations in the line voltage and the ambient conditions, it is essential that the uniformity of response is checked routinely.

Another aspect of the nonuniform response of a scintillation camera is known as edge packing. This is also a manifestation of mispositioning of the counts. It appears as a bright ring around the edge of an image (Fig. 12.8) and is caused by internal reflection of the light at the edge of the crystal and the fact that the PM tubes are present on one side only. As a result, counts coming from near the edges are bunched together. The region of edge packing is never used in clinical studies; it is always masked by a lead ring around the collimator. Thus, the useful field of view is always smaller than the crystal size.

In modern scintillation cameras, the nonuniformity of response has improved considerably by addressing its causes—local variations in the amount of light transmitted to a PM tube and the nonlinear response of the X,Y pulses due to slightly different PM gains. These nonlinearities are very carefully measured, and from these measurements, a correction matrix formed. This correction matrix then appropriately repositions on line all the subsequent counts detected by the camera using a microprocessor. As a result of these corrections, the uniformity of the scintillation camera has improved tremendously and is 2% or better in the useful field of view (Fig. 12.9). Moreover, the electronic components and the PM tubes used in these cameras are more stable than those used in older cameras. Automatic tuning circuits further enhance the stability. Therefore, the new scintillation cameras generally do not require tuning as often; a monthly or

Figure 12.9. Corrected "flood" showing more uniform response of a new scintillation camera with a circular-shaped crystal.

even quarterly interval is adequate for routine maintenance. However, the measurements of the correction matrix are too complicated to be done by in-house personnel; therefore, if a camera detunes significantly from its prescribed limits, a service call is necessary.

The nonuniform transmission of γ-rays by the collimator is tested separately. If it is found unacceptable, the collimator is replaced. Once a satisfactory collimator is found, occasional physical inspection for the presence of dents or unusual marks ensures the integrity of the collimator.

High Count Rate Performance

Because a gamma camera uses a NaI(Tl) crystal to detect γ-rays and to determine the location of γ-ray interaction in the crystal, at high count rates, besides loss of counts due to the finite dead time, mispositioning of counts also takes place. At high count rates, the probability of two γ-rays simultaneously interacting in the crystal (within the dead time of the detector) increases sharply. If one or both γ-rays interact through the photoelectric effect, the total light produced will be more than the light produced if only one γ-ray interacted that way. Therefore, if the pulse-height analyzer (PHA) is set on the photopeak, both of these γ-rays, mimicking as one but with higher energy, will be rejected by the PHA. On the other hand, if both γ-rays interact through the Compton effect and each interaction produces enough light so that the sum of the two is equal to the light produced by the photoelectric interaction of one γ-ray, the two γ-rays, mimicking as one but with correct energy, will be accepted by PHA. However, the location of the interaction will be the mean of the locations of the interactions of the two γ-rays in the displayed image. Thus, a misposition of the count occurs.

The dead time of a scintillation camera is made up of paralyzable and nonparalyzable components. Under ideal conditions, it is between 1 and 2 μsec. However, the dead time of a scintillation camera is a complex function of window width used, scattering material around the source, presence of more than one γ-ray in the emissions of the radionuclide used, and so on. Therefore, it is essential to determine the dead time of a scintillation camera under conditions typically used in clinical situations. In these circumstances, dead time may be as much as

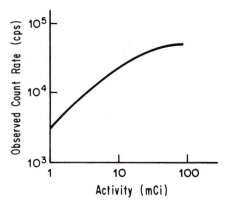

Figure 12.10.   Count rate response of a typical scintillation camera.

10–15 μsec. Count rate performance of a typical scintillation camera is shown in Figure 12.10.

QUALITY CONTROL OF IMAGING DEVICES

Correct interpretation of an image depends on the accuracy of the data in the image. Therefore, it is of utmost importance that nuclear imaging devices operate optimally and reliably. Because these instruments use a variety of electronic components whose response may be affected by changes in line voltage or ambient conditions, the best way to ensure accuracy and reliability of these instruments is through a continuing program of quality control. The quality control procedures are intended to monitor day-to-day variations in some performing characteristics to be alerted, in time, to the malfunction or unacceptable behavior of these instruments. These are semiquantitative procedures and therefore do not measure the operating characteristics of an imaging device accurately or completely. The procedures given in the following sections are brief and therefore illustrate only the important aspects of such an endeavor.

Scintillation Camera

The three most common parameters routinely tested to ensure maximal performance of a scintillation camera are peaking, field uniformity, and spatial resolution.

PEAKING

This test, which is performed every day, ensures that the window of the PHA is correctly set on the desired photopeak. The following steps are involved in peaking a scintillation camera:

1. Place a small radioactive source under the scintillation camera (if the collimator is removed, 100–200 μCi of ^{99m}Tc radioactivity is enough; with the collimator on, 1–2 mCi of ^{99m}Tc radioactivity is preferred).

2. Place the camera in Spectrum mode and set the energy and window for the radionuclide being used (for ^{99m}Tc, 140 keV and 20% window).

3. Observe whether the photopeak is within the window or not. If not, change the high voltage slowly so as to center the photopeak in the window.

4. Take a picture of the spectrum and record the high-voltage setting. The high-voltage setting should not change more than 10% from one day to the next. If the change is greater, investigate the cause because this may lead to a malfunction. At this point, also note any fingerprints, dirt, and so on on the oscilloscope screen.

FIELD UNIFORMITY

This test, which should be performed daily, ensures that the count rate variations in the image of a uniform source are within an acceptable range and the scintillation camera is properly tuned. Because the collimator response is not expected to change unless there is evidence of physical damage, only the intrinsic field uniformity is checked. The following steps are involved:

1. Remove the collimator and move the detector head 4–5 feet above the floor.

2. Place a 100- to 200-μCi small volume (0.2 mL) source of ^{99m}Tc on the floor (use absorbent paper under the source to avoid contamination of the floor).

3. Set the preset count of 10^6 counts for a small field of view and 2×10^6 counts for a large field on the view scintillation camera.

4. Adjust the display oscilloscope intensity to the 10^6 or 2×10^6 count level depending on the type of scintillation camera.

5. Turn the scintillation camera on and record the image.

The resultant image is visually evaluated for uniformity, image shape (it should be a nice circle), and other artifacts. Variations greater than ±10% are easily detectable in the image and are unacceptable. On the older type of scintillation camera with uniformity correction, two images are recorded, one with the microprocessor off and the other with the microprocessor on.

SPATIAL RESOLUTION (INTRINSIC)

Because measurement of the two quantitative indices of spatial resolution, MTF and FWHM, is time-consuming, a semiquantitative evaluation using a 90° quadrant bar phantom is performed. The phantom consists of four sets of parallel lead bars arranged in four quadrants of a Lucite holder as shown in Figure 12.11. The spacings and width of the lead bars vary between each quadrant but are the same within each quadrant. The smallest spacing is chosen to be smaller than the spatial resolution of the scintillation camera. The procedure for evaluation of the intrinsic spatial resolution is identical to that of field uniformity (steps 1–5) except, under step 1, after removing the collimator, the bar phantom is attached in front of the crystal of the scintillation camera. The resultant image is inspected for the separation of the finest bar spacing and linearity of the bars. The recommended frequency for this test is weekly.

Figure 12.11.   A 90° quadrant, parallel lead bar, phantom used for quality control of the spatial resolution of a scintillation camera.

Key Points

1. Spatial resolution and sensitivity are important in assessing performance of a scintillation camera.

2. Spatial resolution is measured either as a full width at half maximum (FWHM) of a point-spread function or in terms of modulation transfer function (MTF).

3. Sensitivity is measured for a point, line, or plane source.

4. Resolution and sensitivity are inversely related.

5. Intrinsic spatial resolution and sensitivity of a scintillation camera depend on the thickness of the crystal and the energy of the γ-ray.

6. Collimator spatial resolution and sensitivity depend on the size of the holes in the collimator and the thickness of the collimator.

7. Collimator resolution degrades with an increase in distance of the source from the collimator.

8. Scintillation camera position-determining circuit produces a nonuniform image of a uniform radionuclidic distribution. To reduce the nonuniformity, on-line correction modules are provided on scintillation cameras. With these modules, typical uniformity is in the range of $\pm 2\%$.

9. Dead time affects the performance of a scintillation camera at high count rates, typically exceeding 20,000 counts per second.

10. Daily uniformity and weekly spatial resolution tests are recommended for quality control of a scintillation camera.

Questions

1. The spatial resolution and sensitivity of a scintillation camera are 10 mm and 50,000 cpm/μCi, respectively. What will be the sensitivity of this camera if a new collimator with 5 mm spatial resolution is used instead?

2. Why are there so many indices of spatial resolution? Give the best application for each of them.

3. Determine the overall spatial resolution of a scintillation camera if the spatial resolution of the collimator is 10 mm and the intrinsic spatial resolution is (a) 10 mm, (b) 5 mm, and (c) 1 mm.

4. Why is about 1 inch of crystal at the edge not usable for imaging in a scintillation camera?

5. In addition to the expected loss of counts, what problem does the dead time of a scintillation camera cause that does not occur in other counting situations?

6. How often (daily, weekly, or yearly) should the following parameters of a scintillation camera be checked? (a) Energy spatial resolution, (b) uniformity, (c) spatial resolution, (d) sensitivity, and (e) energy calibration.

13 Detectability or Final Contrast in an Image

The primary goal in imaging is to detect the smallest possible localized or focal abnormalities (lesions) that may be present in an organ. Because of practical limitations, however, it is not possible to attain this goal. There is a lower limit of detectability below which a lesion cannot be visualized. This limit is determined by a number of parameters discussed below.

OBJECT CONTRAST

The main purpose of any imaging device is to record the details of an object faithfully in its image. What do we mean by the details of an object? These are the spatial variations of a given parameter such as light intensity in photography, transmitted x-ray intensity in diagnostic radiology, and the concentration of radioactivity in scanning. Such a parameter, in the language of the physicist, is known as object contrast and is most important in the detectability of a lesion. In nuclear medicine, the object contrast is created in the organ of interest by the use of radiopharmaceuticals that either selectively localize in the abnormal tissue as compared with the normal tissue, or vice versa. In either case, the higher the variation between the concentration of radioactivity in the normal and abnormal tissue, the easier it is to detect an abnormality. Therefore, radiopharmaceuticals that produce greater contrast in the lesion have better detectability than those that produce smaller contrast.

For quantitative purposes, we may define the object contrast, C_0, as follows:

$$C_0 = \frac{\text{(Concentration in abnormal tissue} - \text{Concentration in normal tissue)}}{\text{Concentration in normal tissue}}$$

When there is no differential (variation) between the concentration of radioactivity in the abnormal and normal tissue, $C_0 = 0$ (i.e., there is no contrast). Such a radiopharmaceutical producing zero object contrast will be of no use in the detection of abnormal lesions. When the concentration of the radioactivity is higher in the abnormal area than that of the normal area, then $C_0 > 0$, and the radiopharmaceutical produces a positive contrast.

For example, radiopharmaceuticals currently used for brain scanning produce positive contrast, with values of C_0 generally ranging from 15 to 25. In cases where there is less radioactivity in a lesion than in normal tissue, radiopharmaceuticals produce a negative contrast ($C_0 < 0$). The value of C_0 for negative contrast cannot be increased more than -1, a value indicating almost no radioactivity in the lesion. For example, radiocolloids used for liver scanning are preferentially localized in normal tissue with almost no radioactivity in the abnormal lesions. Because radiopharmaceuticals producing positive contrast can achieve higher contrast values ($C_0 \geq 1$) than those producing negative contrast, the former potentially have far better detectability than the latter.

SPATIAL RESOLUTION AND SENSITIVITY OF AN IMAGING DEVICE

An imaging device, such as a scintillation camera, registers the details of the distribution of a radionuclide as a photographic camera records the details of an object or scene. In both cases, a physical device is used to form an image of an object. This is true, in fact, of any imaging process using such diverse instruments as an electron microscope, telescope, or x-ray tube. In all cases, the aim is to reproduce exactly the object contrast in the image.

Unfortunately, no imaging device is capable of reproducing all the details of an object in an image, and a certain loss of detail (object contrast) is inevitable. The parameter of an imaging device that characterizes the extent of the loss of object contrast or measures the faithfulness or the fidelity for reproduction of object contrast is called spatial resolution. An imaging device that possesses better spatial resolution is capable of reproducing finer details of an object (smaller object contrasts) and is able to detect smaller lesions than an imaging device with a poorer spatial resolution. Therefore, the spatial resolution of an imager is an important parameter that strongly influences the detectability of a lesion.

What limits the spatial resolution of an imaging device? Theoretically, there are no limitations in designing a scanner with fine spatial resolution capabilities. The limitations arise from the two practical constraints: the radiation dose to the patient must be kept low and the time of scanning should be reasonably short.

The effect of these two restrictions is to limit the number of γ-rays that can be detected and displayed in an image. As we see in the following section, the total number of γ-rays (photons) in an image is also an important parameter affecting the detectability of a lesion. To obtain a given number of photons in an image within a limited time, therefore, the imaging device should possess high sensitivity. The sensitivity of an imaging device is a measure of its ability to detect γ-rays efficiently. A more sensitive device will require a shorter interval of time to detect the same number of γ-rays than a less sensitive device.

Unfortunately, the sensitivity of an imaging device is related as the inverse square to its spatial resolution (see Chapter 12). Therefore, an imaging device with a spatial resolution better by a factor of 2 than a given imaging device will have a fourfold loss of sensitivity. This loss of sensitivity theoretically necessitates either a fourfold increase in the scanning or imaging time or a fourfold increase in the radiation dose to the patient. In actuality, the cost to improve the spatial resolution by a factor of 2 will be more than fourfold, as will be seen in the following section.

STATISTICAL NOISE OR INFORMATION DENSITY

For reproducing the details of an object, even with high contrast, an imaging device with good spatial resolution is not, in itself, enough. The human eye is capable of seeing minute details of a well-lit object but fails to perceive even large objects in a dark room. Hence, the amount of available light (number of photons) is another important parameter affecting the visualization of the details or contrast of an object.

This point is strikingly demonstrated in Figure 13.1, showing six photographs of a girl taken in succession with increasing numbers of total photons. With a smaller number of photons, only large details with high contrast are visible. As the number of photons increases, finer details of the object become visible in the image. In other words, the number of photons needed to visualize a given detail in an object is related to its contrast in the object. This relationship between the number of photons and the object contrast is not limited only to photography but is a generalized phenomenon of any imaging process.

Consequently, the net contrast in an image (it is the contrast in the image that allows us to determine the presence of a lesion) is derived from two components: the finite spatial resolution of the imaging device and the number of photons that make up the image. The latter component determines statistical noise in the image. In a well-lit object (a large number of photons), the limiting factor for reproducing the object contrast is essentially the spatial resolution of the imaging device, whereas in a dark room (hardly any photons), the limiting factor is the statistical noise in the image. In a moderately lit room (a limited number of photons), the final contrast in the image is determined by both.

In nuclear medicine, the statistical noise of an image is related to information density, which is defined as the number of γ-rays detected per cm^2 of an object. If we multiply the information density by the area of the object, we obtain the average number of photons in an image. When performing a scan with a rectilinear scanner, it is convenient to set the information density; in the scintillation camera, it is easier to set the total number of photons. In both cases, the statistical noise can be reduced by increasing either the information density or the total number of photons in the image. The statistical noise or error of N counts in an image equals to $\sqrt{N}$ (p. 26). Because the total number of photons or information density needed to visualize a lesion depends on its contrast in the object, an information density of approximately 1000 counts/cm^2 of the organ (or approximately 300,000 counts in routine brain scans) is generally accepted as an optimum value for currently available imagers. Use of information densities much lower than this value may cause borderline lesions (with low contrast) to be overlooked. On the other hand, increasing the information density higher than this value will not significantly affect the detectability because, at this level, the limiting factor for detectability is the resolution of the imaging device.

Figure 13.1. Photographs taken under identical conditions except for variations in the total amount of light (number of photons). As the number of photons increases, greater detail is visible. A photographic camera possesses fine spatial resolution, yet without an adequate number of photons, that resolution is useless in providing the finer details in an object. (Reprinted by permission from Rose A. Quantum and noise limitations of the visual process. J Optic Soc Am 1953;43:715.)

In the future, if imaging devices with improved spatial resolution but without any loss of sensitivity become available, higher information density will have to be used. For example, an improvement in spatial resolution by a factor of 2 will necessitate an increase in information density approximately by a factor of 4. For the present day imaging devices, however, when we couple this with the fact that improving the spatial resolution will reduce the sensitivity by a factor of 4, we are talking about a factor of roughly 16; that is, an improvement in the lower limit of detectability by a factor of 2 using present day imaging devices and radiopharmaceuticals will lengthen the time of the study approximately 16 times.

PROJECTION OF VOLUME DISTRIBUTION INTO AREAL DISTRIBUTION

An imaging device, such as a gamma camera, in essence integrates the radioactivity present in the third dimension (depth) of an organ. The result of such an integration (i.e., the weighted sum of radioactivity with depth) is to degrade the detectability of a lesion by lowering the object contrast (see Figure 13.2 for a hypothetical situation).

COMPTON SCATTERING OF γ-RAYS

As explained in Chapter 10, a γ-ray originating outside the field of view of a collimator can still reach the radiation detector as a result of Compton scattering. The effect of such scattering is to reduce the object contrast and therefore to degrade the detectability of a lesion. Pulse-height selection used to discriminate against scattered γ-rays has proven quite effective in restoring some of the object contrast lost as a result of Compton scattering. However, because the energy resolution of a NaI(Tl) detector is not very high, a certain amount of object contrast is still lost. Also, as one narrows the window to reject the unwanted (scattered) counts, some good counts are also rejected. Therefore, too narrow a window may improve the image contrast somewhat, but it will be at the cost of sensitivity. This will not be the case for detectors with better energy resolution, such as Ge(Li) detectors. However, it has other shortcomings, as pointed out in Chapter 8.

ATTENUATION

Because attenuation of γ-rays by the tissue of distribution and by the overlying tissue reduces the number of γ-rays reaching a scanner, such a reduction adversely affects the detectability of a lesion. As a result, lesions that are on the surface of an organ are easier to detect than those lying deep within the organ.

MOTION OF THE OBJECT

Motion of the patient or the organ (particularly the liver, lung, and heart, which can move as much as 2 cm) also affects the detectability of a lesion in scanning. The effect of motion in an object is to reduce the object contrast, which then results in a diminished contrast in the image. By using a computer with a scintillation camera, it is feasible to eliminate some loss of object contrast due to motion. Because the clinical usefulness of such a procedure, compared with the time and effort involved, has not been convincingly established, we do not go into the details of this method.

DISPLAY PARAMETERS

The ability to visualize an abnormality is also affected by the display parameters, such as exposure settings, the type of film used, Hurter-Driffield (H-D) curve of the film, and so on. For the proper display, the count rate variations of interest should

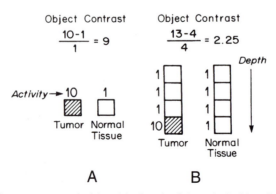

Figure 13.2.   Loss of object contrast as a result of the weighted sum in relation to depth of the radioactivity in routine area scanning. In this example, as a result of summation, a tumor with a contrast of 9 appears to have a contrast of 2.25 only. Here, equal weight is given to each box; in actual scanning, their exact contribution to summation will depend on the variation of the sensitivity with depth.

match the H-D curve's useful latitude (between points A and B of Figure 10.7).

OBSERVER VARIATIONS

In noise-limited images, the detectability of a lesion is also dependent on the observer (in this case, the nuclear medicine physician). Because in noise-limited images, a decision has to be made whether a given lesion is a manifestation of noise or not (false or true), such a decision may vary from observer to observer. Observer variation can be studied using what is known as receiver operated characteristic curves.

Key Points

1. Detectability of a lesion is a complex function of several parameters, which may depend on the patient, the scintillation camera, or the imaging technique.

2. Object contrast depends on the patient (radiopharmaceutical distribution, scatter, and attenuation).

3. Spatial resolution and sensitivity depend on the scintillation camera.

4. The number of counts detected and therefore the statistical noise in the image depends on the technique. Display parameters used also depend on the technique.

Questions

1. What should be the minimum contrast between a normal liver and a metastatic lesion (2 cm in diameter) for it to be visualized (at 99% confidence level) when the information density of a liver scintigram is 1000 counts/cm^2?

2. Do the radiopharmaceuticals designed to study blood flow in the brain have more or less contrast than the radiopharmaceuticals designed for tumor detection? Which of the two has better detectability?

3. Disregarding the consideration of cost, suggest a way to increase the sensitivity and therefore the detectability of a scintillation camera.

4. Why is the detectability for tumor detection in brain similar in nuclear medicine and computed tomography when the resolution for computed tomography is an order of magnitude higher than that in nuclear medicine?

14   Emission Computed Tomography

Area scanning or imaging, even with multiple views, does not provide accurate three-dimensional information concerning radionuclide distribution. Also, because two-dimensional imaging more or less integrates the information from the third dimension (depth), it results in lower contrast of lesions (see Chapter 13). With the advent and success of computed tomography (CT) in diagnostic radiology, similar concepts and techniques have been applied in nuclear medicine as emission computed tomography (ECT). Tomography, in general, is divided into two categories, transverse and longitudinal. It is the transverse tomography that has found success in routine clinical and research use. Transverse tomography can be performed with radionuclides emitting single photons (x- or γ-rays) or with radionuclides emitting positrons. Transverse tomography with single photon emitters is commonly known as SPECT (or SPET), whereas with positron emitters it is known as PET (or, rarely, PECT). Longitudinal tomography is performed with single photons only.

This chapter describes the principle of transverse tomography, instruments commonly used for SPECT and PET, and the relative merits of the two types. The mathematical techniques used in reconstruction of a tomogram are highly sophisticated and are beyond the scope of this book. Therefore, I limit myself to a phenomenologic description only. Longitudinal tomography is also discussed briefly.

PRINCIPLES OF TRANSVERSE TOMOGRAPHY

In its simplest form, a detector acquires data from a thin axial section containing radioactivity by linear scanning from multiple directions around the cross section, as shown in Figure 14.1. In its complex form, mainly to reduce the data acquisition time, data may be acquired from multiple thin cross sections and multiple directions simultaneously by using a large number of detectors or a scintillation camera. In either case, the principle of transverse tomography is the same and consists of two steps: acquisition of

linear projection data of a thin cross section from multiple directions and reconstruction of the cross section or cross sections from these data.

Considerations in Data Acquisition

PIXEL WIDTH, MATRIX, AND NUMBER OF PROJECTIONS

Let us consider a simple case where a single detector linearly scans a cross section from many directions. Let us also assume that as the detector moves from one position to the next along a line, it receives counts from N columns that are perpendicular to the direction of a scan and chosen to be equally spaced. This is shown in Figure 14.2 for the two positions of the detector in two different linear scans. Two columns perpendicular to each other have only a small area in common. This area is called a pixel, and the entire cross section can be imagined to consist of these small pixels distributed in a square matrix of size N × N. When scans are performed from different directions, different combinations of pixels, but always perpendicular to the direction of scan, contribute to the counts of the detector at different positions along a scan line. These are called projections of a plane on a line, and the number M of these projections is a critical parameter in the reconstruction of the cross section. For accurate and artifact-free reconstruction, M should be nearly equal to N. From the projection data, the radioactivity of each pixel is computed using the method described in the next section.

Data acquisition with a single detector is very time-consuming. A variety of methods has been developed to reduce the acquisition time or to increase the overall sensitivity. For example, to avoid the linear motion, a linear array of detectors (N) can be used simultaneously to gather data from a projection. This increases sensitivity N-fold compared with a single detector. Further gains can be achieved by using multiple linear arrays gathering data simultaneously from multiple directions as well as from many cross sections. Of course, such an increase in sensitivity is accompanied by an increased complexity and cost of such a device. Sensitivity is the main reason why data acquisition

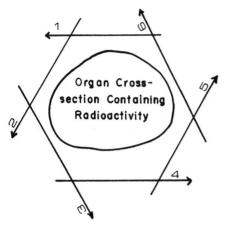

Figure 14.1. Principle of axial tomography. A thin cross section of an organ is scanned from several tangential directions (in this example, six). From these scans, the cross-sectional radioactive distribution is reconstructed, using a variety of superimpositional techniques.

with a scintillation camera for SPECT is routinely used in clinical nuclear medicine.

The number of pixels in a cross section is determined by the number of columns, N, in a scan direction and is simply N × N. In the case of Figure 14.2, this number is 9 × 9 = 81. In a given cross section, the number of pixels and the size of the pixel (Δx) are inversely related. The smaller the pixel size, the larger the number of pixels or matrix size. In actual practice, the matrix size is either 64 × 64 or 128 × 128, resulting in 4096 or 16,384 pixels, respectively. What determines the pixel size is discussed next.

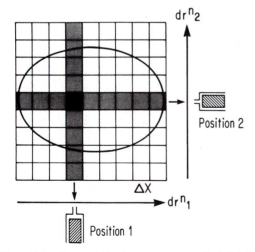

Figure 14.2. Data acquisitions in transverse tomography. dr^{n_1}, dr^{n_2} stand for scan directions 1, 2, ...

PIXEL WIDTH, RESOLUTION, AND SENSITIVITY

Pixel width, Δx, (and therefore the matrix size, N × N, and number of linear projections, M) is an important consideration in data acquisition because it pertains to the amount of time required to complete a scan. Pixel width depends on the resolution obtainable in the tomogram, which in turn depends on the resolution of the collimator used in SPECT or the size of the detector used in PET. A rule of thumb is that the pixel width (Δx) should be less than or equal to the resolution. Thus, in general, improving the resolution necessitates reducing the pixel width, Δx, and vice versa. However, to reduce resolution, one has to reduce the size of the hole in the collimator of the detector (SPECT) or use smaller size detectors (PET), which reduces the sensitivity of the detector. Thus, to achieve the same statistical reliability, one has to increase the time spent at each location. In addition, the reduction in Δx as a result of higher resolution increases the number of pixels, N, along the scan line that necessitates more linear projections, M, from different angles for optimum sampling. This again requires more time. Thus, we face a similar (actually worse) dilemma in transverse tomography as we face in areal scanning, that is, improvement in resolution costs dearly in terms of sensitivity and a compromise has to be made between the two. In CT, where, because of the large number of photons available from an x-ray tube, the typical resolution or pixel size is about 1 mm, the number of linear scans performed is 180 or more. In nuclear medicine, where the available number of photons in a typical cross section is relatively small, typical resolution is in the range of 1 cm and the number of linear scans needed is in the vicinity of 64 (128 for high resolution).

OTHER REQUIREMENTS

Besides the width Δx of the columns, the other important requirements of collimation are

1. An individual detector at a given location picks up counts from only one column (perpendicular to the scan direction);

2. There are no variations in counts detected from a uniform cross section at different locations along scans from multiple directions;

3. The same activity in any pixel in a column contributes equally to the counts at a given location (i.e., the detector response should be uniform with depth);

4. All counts come from only the cross section under consideration and not from adjacent cross sections.

These requirements are not easily achieved in nuclear medicine because of the nature of collimation and attenuation and scatter in the patient, particularly for SPECT as described later.

A major difference between CT and ECT in data acquisition is that in CT, data are acquired within a 180° rotation of linear scans, whereas in SPECT (except for heart studies where 180° is preferable), a complete rotation (360°) of linear scans around the cross section is used.

Reconstruction of the Cross Section

Reconstruction of a cross section from its multiple linear projections around the cross section is a general problem that is encountered in diverse fields. Its solution was provided by Radon as far back as 1917. However, because of the complexity involved in the computations, practical realization of the solution was achieved only in recent years with the advent and easy access to large digital computers. There are a number of mathematical techniques to solve this problem; the most common method is known as filtered back projection, which is a modified form (therefore more accurate) of back projection. Back projection can be easily understood with the help of Figure 14.3.

BACK PROJECTION, A SIMPLE EXPLANATION OF RECONSTRUCTION

Let us consider a simple cross section containing two radionuclide sources as depicted in Figure 14.3a. When data are acquired from this cross section with an appropriate detector and by linear scanning from multiple directions, the responses of the detector are shown as scan 1, scan 2, scan 3, scan 4, and so on. Notice that in this case, the detector receives counts only at one or two discrete locations in each scan, and these locations are determined by the intersection of the scan directions and the perpendicular lines from each source to the scan direction, respectively.

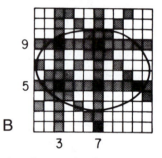

Figure 14.3.   Reconstruction of a cross section using simple back projection method.

In the back projection method of reconstruction, as the name implies, data received at one location of a linear scan is back projected in the column right above that location and so on. Because no prior knowledge exists about which or how many pixels in that column contain radioactivity (actually, that is what we would like to know), one assumes that counts received at that location came in equal amounts from each pixel in that column. This is done in Figure 14.3b. Counts received by the detector in scan 1 at the two locations are distributed equally in the 12 pixels of columns 3 and 7, respectively. When a similar procedure is repeated for other scans (2, 3, 4, etc.), the reconstruction of the cross section is complete. As can be seen, two radioactive sources have been reproduced at the correct locations, although not as point sources but as star patterns. As a result, a number of pixels (shown as shaded) that contained no radioactivity in the original cross section are reconstructed inaccurately as containing small amounts of radioactivity.

FILTERED BACK PROJECTION: ACTUAL STEPS

In a more refined approach, known as filtered back projection, the star artifacts are removed by adding and subtracting fixed fractions of the counts from the column under consideration to several adjacent columns on both sides. When this is done, an accurate and artifact-free reconstruction is obtained. Because data acquired are large and the mathematical operations needed for reconstruction are huge, a large digital computer is essential to store and process the data quickly. In practice, the filtered back reconstruction is performed in frequency or Fourier space (similar to modulation transfer function [MTF] discussed in Chapter 12) where the filter function takes a much simpler form and therefore computations become easier and faster. The following steps are taken:

1. Compute Fourier transform of individual projection data;

2. Multiply it with the filter function;

3. Compute inverse Fourier transform;

4. Back projection to get the cross section.

Filter function is an important parameter in ECT because it affects the noise and resolution characteristics of the reconstruction. A number of filters—ramp, Hanning, Butterworth, Metz—have been used. Of these, Hanning and Butterworth are most common in clinical nuclear medicine.

OTHER METHODS

Besides the filtered back projection, a number of other mathematical methods have been used to reconstruct cross sections from the projection data. Their principal drawback is the computer time needed for reconstruction. However, with the vast improvements in computer data processing speed per unit cost, it is no longer a problem, and these methods may become useful particularly in specific applications. Algebraic reconstruction technique and iterative least-squares technique are two of these methods.

SINGLE-PHOTON EMISSION COMPUTED TOMOGRAPHY
Data Acquisition With a Scintillation Camera

Of the two current approaches for performing SPECT, using either multidetectors or a scintillation camera, the latter is more popular because most of the equipment needed (e.g., a scintillation camera and a computer) is already available in nuclear medicine departments. Additionally, a rotating gantry on which a scintillation camera head can be mounted and a software program to acquire data and reconstruct the cross sections are needed. To reduce the acquisition time further, SPECT systems with two or three scintillation camera heads are preferred.

In this setup (Fig. 14.4), a scintillation camera head (or heads) rotates in a circle around a patient, making a number of stops for a given time to acquire data from multiple directions (64 or 128 in routine procedures). This is a step and shoot data acquisition. No data are gathered during its movement from one position to the next. To avoid this dead time and increase sensitivity further, acquisition protocols have been developed, where data are either gathered continuously (without a stop) or in a combination of the two (continuous + step and shoot). The orbit of detector heads does not have to be circular. Elliptical or body contour orbits, because of their improved sensitivity and resolution characteristics, are now standard features.

Because a scintillation camera acquires data simultaneously from a large area of an organ as opposed to a thin section, data acquired are planar projections of a volume rather than line projections of a cross section. Therefore, it can be easily formatted to produce different cross sections (axial, coronal, sagittal, or oblique) of an organ from just a single acquisition. This is another advantage of a scintillation camera-based SPECT over multidetector-based SPECT systems that presently reproduce only one or two cross sections at a time.

Collimators

For optimal performance of SPECT with a scintillation camera, choice of a collimator is very important. For routine use, a general pur-

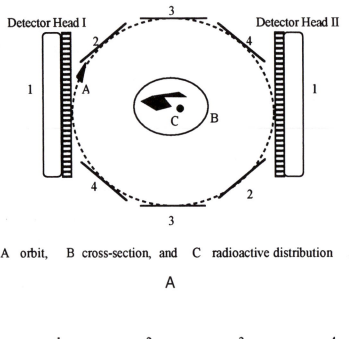

A   orbit,   B   cross-section,   and   C   radioactive distribution

A

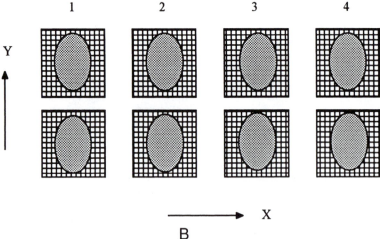

B

Figure 14.4. **(A)** Data acquisition with a dual-head scintillation camera making a circular orbit around a patient containing radioactivity. In this example, four pair of areal projections are acquired. In actual case 32 or 64, such pairs are obtained. **(B)** Corresponding rows in the four pair of images (first row in each image, etc.) represent linear projections for an axial cross section at the level represented by that row. These data are then used in reconstruction of that cross section. The thickness of the cross section can be increased by combining adjacent rows.

pose parallel-hole collimator is preferred. A high resolution parallel-hole collimator may be used in special situations. Special collimators designed for SPECT are also increasingly becoming available. Of these, the so-called fan-beam collimator—parallel holes in one direction and converging holes in the second direction—is finding success because of its improved sensitivity and resolution. However, because the field of view of such a collimator decreases in one direction with depth, caution has to be exercised to avoid artifacts. To reduce scattering and divergence of field view with depth, special collimators with longer holes (thickness L of a collimator) are also being investigated.

Attenuation Correction

The requirement for accurate reconstruction of a cross section—the sensitivity for each pixel in a column is the same and the counts at each location originate only from that column—is not met in SPECT because the γ-rays originating from different pixels pass through different thicknesses of tissues and therefore are attenuated to different degrees. As a result, when reconstruction is done from the data obtained from a cross section of uniform radioactive distribution, it is highly nonuniform. Several methods have been used to solve these problems. These can be classified as analytical or empirical. Analytical methods make some simplifying assumptions about attenuation (e.g., uniformity of attenuating medium) and are incorporated prereconstruction (Sorenson's method), simultaneous with reconstruction (Gulberg's method), or postreconstruction (Chang's method). Of these, the Sorenson and Chang methods are widely available commercially. These methods fail utterly when the attenuating medium is highly inhomogeneous, such as thorax. With empirical methods, the actual attenuation map is obtained by taking multiple transmission scans from multiple projections (similar to a CT). These methods in theory produce the best results but require additional setup and scan time, and exposure to the patient.

Scatter Correction

Compton scattering of γ-rays originating outside the column of interest into the detector and the diverging field of view of a collimator makes it hard to collect data at a given location from one column (and one cross section) only (see Fig. 10.2). As was suggested in Figure 10.2, the best method to reject scattered events is by using either a narrow window or multiple (two or three routinely) windows and subtracting the scattered events.

Resolution Correction

As discussed in Chapter 11, the system resolution of a scintillation camera depends on the depth of the radionuclide source. This is another source of error that has to be corrected if accuracy of SPECT reconstruction is to be further improved. Methods are being developed to correct for this error, and some of these are now available commercially.

Other Requirements or Sources of Error

For accurate reproduction of a radioactive cross section, the following sources of error are unique for a scintillation camera-based SPECT:

1. Center of rotation: Proper alignment of the center of electronic position- (x, y) determining circuit with the center of rotation. In areal imaging, a shift by one or two pixels in the x or y direction is hardly noticeable, but in SPECT, such a misalignment produces recognizable artifacts (e.g., a point source is reconstructed as a ring). Proper alignment can be achieved by placing a point source at the center of rotation, imaging it from two opposite directions, and determining the pixel location of the source in the two images. If these are identical, then there is no need for adjustment and the electronic center is properly aligned with the center of rotation. However, if the pixel location of the source is not identical, these are made identical by electronically off setting X or Y voltage, as the case may be.

2. Uniformity: Uniformity of response of a scintillation camera. This requirement is much more stringent in SPECT than routine imaging because errors propagate rapidly in reconstruction of the image. Although in areal imaging uniformity in the range of ±5% is acceptable, in SPECT it should be under ±2%. As explained earlier (p. 121), newer scintillation cameras are capable of such a performance.

3. Invariance of uniformity at different angles: Because images are acquired at a large number of angles, the uniformity of a scintillation camera should be maintained at each angle. The main reason for changes in the uniformity response at different angles is the change in the photomultiplier (PM) tube gain that occurs when it is oriented at different angles in the earth's magnetic field. In newer cameras where PM tubes are shielded by μ-metal, these effects are reduced considerably.

4. Detector head alignment with the axis of rotation.

Figure 14.5.   Typical SPECT images. (**A**) Sixteen transverse cross sections through the head showing distribution of ^{99m}Tc methylene diphosphonate in head and facial bones, and (**B**) 16 transverse cross sections through the abdomen showing distribution of ^{99m}Tc albumin aggregates in liver and spleen. (Courtesy of Dr. J Sanger, N.Y.U. Medical Center.)

Thus, clinical success of SPECT depends on a stringent quality control program; acquisition of a sufficient number of counts in each image; use of properly designed collimators; and proper correction for attenuation, scatter, and, if possible, for system resolution.

With proper attention to these points, good quality reconstructed SPECT images can be realized routinely in a clinical nuclear medicine department (Fig. 14.5). However, these images, although useful clinically, still fall short where accurate quantitative measurements are required.

POSITRON EMISSION TOMOGRAPHY

Why PET?

Most radionuclides used in nuclear medicine (e.g., ^{99m}Tc, ^{67}Ga, ^{201}Tl) are not isotopes of physiologically important elements such as hydrogen, carbon, nitrogen, or oxygen. The only γ-emitting isotopes of these elements are actually positron emitters (^{11}C, ^{13}N, and ^{15}O) and have short half-lives (in minutes). Fluorine-18, which is also a positron emitter, can replace hydrogen in many important biological molecules without changing their function significantly; for example, ^{18}F-deoxyglucose (^{18}FDG) can be used to measure glucose utilization rate by a tissue such as brain. Because of the potential of positron-emitting radionuclides for measurement of important physiologic parameters noninvasively, there is a great interest in these radionuclides, even when their short half-life poses a tremendous hardship in the routine availability of radiopharmaceuticals labeled with these radionuclides. Some of these problems in developing short-lived radiopharmaceuticals for use with PET have been recently mitigated with the introduction of turnkey cyclotrons and automated radiopharmaceutical production. In addition, several generator systems specifically for PET use are commercially available (e.g., ^{68}Ge-^{68}Ga and ^{82}Sr-^{82}Rb).

Principles of PET

Positron-emitting radionuclides as such do not emit γ-rays, but when an emitted positron has lost its energy by interaction with surrounding medium within a short distance of the site of emission, it annihilates by combining with an electron, and two γ-rays with energies of 511 keV each are produced simultaneously. Such a pair of γ-rays produced by annihilation of a positron always travel in opposite (180° apart) directions. In PET or positron scanning, these two γ-rays are used in a coincidence mode where both γ-rays are detected by a pair of NaI(Tl) detectors simultaneously, as shown in Figure 14.6. Two small NaI(Tl) detectors face each other on either side of a radioactive organ. Output of each detector is then relayed to a coincidence circuit to determine whether the output of each detector originated simultaneously or within a short time of each other ($< 10^{-9}$ seconds). As can be seen, simultaneous detection of the two annihilation γ-rays defines a nice field of view (a cylindrical column as opposed to a cone for a single detector with a collimator) uniquely without the aid of a collimator. One complication that defeats this function arises because of the accidental coincidences that occur from the accidental interactions of two unrelated (not from the same annihilation, e.g., in Figure 14.6, if the two annihilations 4 and 5 occur by chance at the same time, then this will produce a coincidence, although it will not be from one annihilation) rays. Accidental coincidences can be easily controlled as well as corrected. Also note that in this setup, the sensitivity and resolution in the field of view of such a pair of detectors does not vary with the location of radioactive source in its field of view. This, as was stated earlier, is an important requirement for ECT that is difficult to achieve in SPECT but is fulfilled easily in PET. Also, the two annihilation γ-rays taken together pass through the same thickness of tissue irrespective of location of the annihilation in the field of view of the detector pair. Therefore, it is much easier and more accurate to correct for attenuation. Again, this is one more advantage over SPECT.

PET Instrumentation

To perform PET, one can acquire data from a thin cross section with a pair of detectors by linearly scanning a cross section from multiple directions. However, the sensitivity of such a device will be low. To increase the sensitivity, multiple pairs of detectors either in a ring or a hexagonal array are used in commercially available systems, as shown in Figure 14.7. To in-

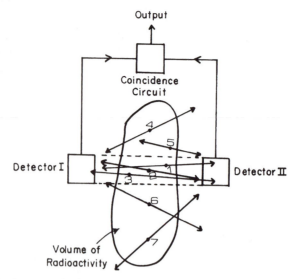

Figure 14.6. Coincidence mode of scanning a distribution of a positron-emitting radionuclide. Only those annihilation photons produced in the volume shown by the dotted lines (e.g., 1, 2, and 3) have a chance of arriving at the two detectors simultaneously. Annihilation photons produced at locations outside this volume (e.g., 4, 5, 6, and 7) will not reach the two detectors simultaneously. Thus, such a pair of detectors measures the radioactivity, without the use of a collimator, of a small volume only. By moving such a pair of detectors over the organ of interest, a scan of the radioactive distribution is produced.

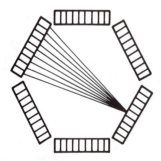

Figure 14.7. Circular or hexagonal arrays of detectors for simultaneous collection of data from various directions in a PET imager. Each detector in the array or ring is in coincidence with a large number of detectors on its opposite side. Here, only one detector is shown in coincidence with several detectors on the opposite side.

crease the sensitivity of these devices, more than one array or ring is sometimes used to acquire data from multiple cross sections simultaneously. Bismuth germanate crystals, which have a higher intrinsic efficiency for 511-keV γ-rays, are used instead of NaI(Tl) crystals. The resolution of these devices can approach 5 mm.

Because PET, in addition to the instrumentation just described, uses short-lived radionuclides, a small on-site cyclotron is needed, which makes this technique quite expensive. As a result, only a small number of medical centers are presently exploring the clinical potential of this technique.

HIGH-ENERGY SPECT AND PET WITH A SCINTILLATION CAMERA

The success of PET, particularly of ^{18}FDG in brain, has inspired the possible use of the scintillation camera with the positron-emitting radionuclides in a single detection mode (511-keV γ-rays without coincidence). To accomplish this, one needs high-energy collimators and high quality of shielding of the NaI(Tl) detector. Routine areal projection or SPECT can be performed.

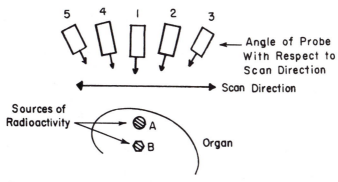

Figure 14.8. Longitudinal tomography using a rectilinear scanner. An organ is scanned several times in a plane parallel to the plane of interest in the organ with the detector head inclined at various angles. The superimposition of these scans in a specified manner produces the tomogram of the plane of interest.

However, the sensitivity is poor compared with either PET or routine ^{99m}Tc imaging. Another variation of the same theme is the coincidence detection of positron-emitting radionuclides with a dual-head scintillation camera. These methods are suited for occasional use of positron-emitting radionuclides and come nowhere near the performance of a dedicated PET instrument.

LONGITUDINAL TOMOGRAPHY

In longitudinal tomography, an organ is scanned with the detector head moving in a plane parallel to the plane of interest in the organ. A number of scans are obtained from multiple directions in that plane (plane of detector head motion) by angling the detector head of a rectilinear scanner. These scans are then super-imposed in such a way that best resolution is achieved for a given plane in the organ (Fig. 14.8). Although superimposition can be achieved photographically, use of a computer for this purpose is faster and more reliable. Longitudinal tomography can also be performed with an Anger camera using a collimator with slanted holes and imaging the organ from different directions by rotating the collimator accordingly (Fig. 14.9). A recent addition to this type of tomography is a seven pinhole collimator, which produces seven images of an organ taken from seven different angles. From these images, different planes of the organ are reconstructed. Longitudinal tomography has met little clinical success primarily because it does not remove the radioactivity present above or below the plane of interest but only blurs that information.

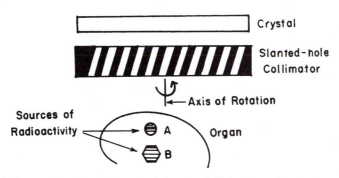

Figure 14.9. Longitudinal tomography using an Anger camera. A slanted parallel-hole collimator is used to image an organ. By rotating this collimator along the axis passing through the center of the collimator and perpendicular to it, multiple images of the organ are obtained from many angles. The reconstruction of the plane of interest is then achieved by superimposition of these images again in a specified manner.

Key Points

1. Emission computed tomography determines a radionuclidic distribution in a tissue cross section such as axial, sagittal, or coronal.

2. Linear projection data are collected from multiple directions.

3. The cross section is then reconstructed from these data using mathematical algorithms. Of these, the most common is filtered back projection.

4. Single-photon emission computed tomography (SPECT) is easily performed with a scintillation camera attached to a rotating gantry and a digital computer.

5. Two problems that make quantification difficult in SPECT are attenuation and scatter. Recent methods of dealing with these two problems—measurement of attenuation with transmission and scatter correction with triple windows—have reduced the quantification errors significantly.

6. Positron emission tomography (PET) uses positron annihilation radiations (two 511-keV γ-rays traveling in opposite directions) in coincidence mode to collimate (electronic collimation as opposed to mechanical collimators). In coincidence mode, attenuation and scatter can be dealt with easily and reasonably accurately. This leads to accurate quantification of in vivo radioactivity by PET.

Questions

1. Is it essential to acquire data from all sides (360° angle) for accurate reconstruction in SPECT? Can it be less than 180°?

2. What is the primary benefit in using a dual- or triple-head scintillation camera in SPECT? What additional problems, if any, do these entail?

3. Why is quality control important in SPECT?

4. What two factors make quantitation with SPECT less accurate than PET?

5. Why is the resolving time of a coincidence circuit an important parameter in a PET scanner?

15   Biological Effects of Radiation and Risk Evaluation From Radiation Exposure

Interaction of radiation with biological systems results in a variety of biological changes that can be either deleterious or benign. These changes may become evident immediately or may take years or generations before being manifested. In general, the probability of occurrence and the type and severity of these changes depend on many factors, some related to radiation and its characteristics and others to biological characteristics of the system. Because a detailed account of these changes and the factors affecting them fall under the discipline of radiation biology, the discussion here is limited to only those aspects of radiation biology that are essential for an assessment of the possible dangers in the use of radiation as these relate to nuclear medicine.

MECHANISM OF BIOLOGICAL DAMAGE

Manifestation of bioinjury due to radiation is always preceded by a complex series of physiochemical events, as shown in Figure 15.1.

The first step in this series of events is the deposition of energy by radiation in the form of ionization and excitation of some atoms or molecules of the biological system as was explained in Chapter 6. This generally lasts about 10^{-12} seconds or less.

The second step, which may last from 10^{-12} to 10^{-3} seconds, is the transfer of energy either to neighboring molecules (intermolecular) or, quite often, within the molecule itself (intramolecular) to form various short-lived and chemically active species known as free radicals (atomic or molecular entities with an unpaired electron and shown by a dot to the right side of the chemical symbol). Because water (H_2O) constitutes 75–85% of the mass of a living system, most ionization is produced in water, and the two most common radicals formed are H· and OH·.

In the next stage, which may last from milliseconds to several seconds, the free radicals react either among themselves or, more significantly, with other important biomolecules (e.g.,

DNA, RNA) to produce alterations in them. Reactions of H· and OH· radicals with important biological molecules cause most radiation damage observed in living systems.

The final step (i.e., the expression of the biological alteration produced in the previous stage) is the biological damage that is tied to the fate of these altered biomolecules. Eventual biological damage may be manifested within a short time or may be delayed up to several generations, depending on the type and function of these altered molecules and on the repair capacity of the irradiated biological system.

FACTORS AFFECTING BIOLOGICAL DAMAGE

Biological damage (or effect) of a system caused by radiation depends on the following factors.

Radiation Dose

Any biological effect of radiation, whether deleterious or benign, strongly depends on the radiation dose. Generally, more effects, and more serious effects, are produced by high than low doses. The exact relationship of the dose to the effect produced, however, depends on the nature of the effect. For example, the dose-effect relationship for the induction of cancer differs from that causing genetic mutation. Depending on the dose-effect relationship, radiation effects are termed as stochastic or deterministic. In stochastic effects, the probability of occurrence and not the severity of the effect depends on the radiation dose. Two important examples are induction of cancer and genetic damage, where the probabilities of induction are a function of radiation dose but their severity is not. Stochastic effects do not have a threshold, a dose level below which the probability of occurrence is zero. Therefore, in radiation protection, where stochastic effects are of major concern, a common assumption is made that states that risk from radiation is directly proportional to dose without

Figure 15.1.   Various stages in the development of bioinjury caused by high-energy radiation.

a threshold. This assumption forms the basis of the so-called ALARA principle of radiation protection, discussed in Chapter 16.

In deterministic effects, on the other hand, the severity of effect depends on the radiation dose and has a threshold, a dose below which no effect is observed. Two examples of deterministic effects of radiation are production of cataracts and erythema.

Dose Rate

In the case of low linear energy transfer (LET) radiations, if the same dose is delivered to two identical biological systems, one with a short duration (high dose rate) and the other over a longer period of time (low dose rate), the biological responses of the two systems will differ. High dose rates are more damaging than low dose rates.

LET or Type of Radiation

Higher LET (see p. 52) radiations (α particles and protons) per unit of absorbed dose produce

greater damage in a biological system than lower LET radiations (electrons and γ- and x-rays). The relative biological effectiveness (RBE) of a radiation for producing a given effect in a biological system under the same conditions is defined as follows:

$$RBE = \frac{\text{Dose of a standard (x-ray) radiation needed to produce a biological effect}}{\text{Dose of a second radiation needed to produce the same biological effect}}$$

For example, the RBE of 10-MeV neutrons for killing cells is about 10. In other words, 10-MeV neutrons are 10 ten times more effective at cell killing than x-rays (generally, 250-kVp x-rays are used as a reference). The "quality factor," Q, and radiation weighting factor, w_R, discussed in next section are estimated from the RBE of a radiation.

Type of Tissue

Biological response of a system varies widely depending on the type of tissue (e.g., liver, bone marrow, or nerve tissue) involved. Given the same radiation dose and dose rate, bone marrow is much more sensitive than nerve tissue to certain types of radiation damage.

Amount of Tissue

Injury to a biological system also depends on the amount of tissue irradiated. For example, a mammal can tolerate a much higher dose to a part of the body than irradiation of the total body.

Rate of Cell Turnover

The rate of cell turnover in tissues is deemed to affect the latent period for the expression of tissue damage. For tissues with a rapid cell turnover (bone marrow), damage appears earlier than for a slow cell turnover (liver).

Biological Variation

The response of a biological system, even with all other factors constant, may vary enormously even among closely related individuals. One person may survive a total body dose of 400 rad (cGy), whereas a dose of only 200 rad (cGy) in another person may be lethal.

Chemical Modifiers

The presence of certain chemicals is known to modify the response of a biological system to radiation. Substances that make biological systems more radioresistant are called radioprotectors. A good example of a radioprotector is the protein, cysteine. Substances that make biological systems more radiosensitive are called radiosensitizers. An example of a radiosensitizer is molecular oxygen. For a radioprotector or radiosensitizer to have any effect, it must be present in the biological system during irradiation.

BIOLOGICAL EFFECT, EQUIVALENT DOSE, AND DOSE EQUIVALENT

Because biological effects, in addition to being dependent on dose, are modified by many factors, how do we take into account some of these factors when comparing the radiation risk from radiation doses delivered under a variety of conditions? Two advisory groups, the International Council on Radiation Protection and the National Council on Radiation Protection (NCRP), perform this task by considering the most recent scientific data and issuing periodic recommendations on the issues related to radiation protection. These recommendations are subsequently adopted, with minor variations, as rules or regulations by appropriate regulatory agencies. In the United States, the Nuclear Regulatory Commission (NRC) serves this purpose, and its rules and regulations are published in the Code of Federal Regulations under Title 10.

When comparing radiation risks, one factor, type of radiation, has been explicitly considered. This is incorporated by the NCRP in the definition of a new term, "equivalent dose." The NRC still uses the old term "dose equivalent," which is slightly different as noted below. Tissue sensitivity and related aspects are considered later in this chapter.

Equivalent Dose

Because biological effects per unit absorbed dose in a tissue T are dependent on the type of radiation (x- and γ-ray versus proton and α particle), a weighting factor, w_R, is defined for each type of radiation to account for these differences.

The weighted dose is called equivalent dose. To distinguish it from the absorbed dose, D, it is given in rem in conventional units and sievert (Sv) in SI units, denoted by the letter H. Thus,

$$H \text{ (rem or Sv)} = w_R \times D \text{ (rad or Gy)} \quad [1]$$

Luckily for radiations used in radiology or nuclear medicine (x- and γ-rays, electrons and positrons), w_R equals 1. Therefore, dose (D) and equivalent dose (H) are the same in amount but different in units, rem versus rad (Gy versus Sv). Consequently, all doses calculated in Chapter 7 can be easily converted into equivalent doses by simply changing the units from rad to rem (Gy to Sv). For neutrons and α particles, w_R has a much higher value (10-20), but these do not concern us here.

Dose Equivalent

Dose equivalent is used in NRC regulations and defined by an equation similar to equation (1) above except that instead of a radiation weighting factor, w_R, a radiation quality factor, Q_R, is used. For radiations used in nuclear medicine, Q_R is also one. Another difference is that, in the above equation, D is an average dose to a tissue, whereas dose equivalent is computed from dose to a point in the tissue. For all practical purposes in nuclear medicine, these two terms are interchangeable.

DELETERIOUS EFFECTS IN HUMANS

Deleterious effects in humans may be acute (mainly deterministic) or late (mainly stochastic). Acute effects are manifested within a short period after irradiation and range from transient nausea and vomiting to death. Late effects may take as long as several generations for eventual manifestation. These include stochastic effects, for example, induction of cancer and leukemia, birth defects and other abnormalities in the offspring of the irradiated person (genetic damage), and nonstochastic effects, for example, cataracts, shortening of the overall life span, and production of temporary or permanent sterility in an individual.

Acute Effects

These are generally produced when the radiation dose is high and delivered to a large part of the body in a short duration. Five clinically distinct stages can be identified as the radiation dose is progressively increased: no effect, mild damage to bone marrow, severe damage to bone marrow and mild damage to the gastrointestinal tract, severe damage to the gastrointestinal tract, and damage to the central nervous system. Table 15.1 lists the radiation doses and the typical symptoms produced for the four stages.

Late Effects

Late effects may occur in cases where acute reactions are minimal (i.e., when the radiation dose to the total body is low or only part of the body is involved in the irradiation). In diagnostic uses of radiation, whether in radiology or nuclear medicine, the range of radiation doses generally delivered to a patient falls in this category. Therefore, the dose-effect relationship of late effects is of special interest.

Regrettably, precise information about the risks involving low radiation doses is difficult to obtain for the following reasons. First, the probability of occurrence of any late effect after low doses is small. Therefore, to perform statistically valid studies, large populations have to be considered. In practice, this is difficult to implement. Second, the occurrence of a latent period in the expression of late effects requires a long follow-up (10 years or more). Finally, late effects of radiation also occur naturally and more frequently than those caused by low doses of radiation. Because accurate information is lacking on the natural frequency of these effects, it is difficult to estimate the influence (increase or decrease) of low radiation doses. In addition, the frequency of natural occurrence is influenced by

many complex factors such as age, sex, genetic history, geography, and various environmental and socioeconomic factors.

Despite these obstacles, a good estimation has been made of the risks to a person or a population exposed to low radiation doses. Most information in this regard is derived from two sources: extrapolation from experiments conducted on laboratory animals (e.g., mice) and retrospective studies of the victims of the atomic bomb explosions in Nagasaki and Hiroshima, the inhabitants of Bikini and other Pacific islands who were exposed to radiation as a result of fallout, persons irradiated for medical reasons, and occupational workers such as uranium mine workers and radiation workers (e.g., radiologists). Two scientific committees, the United Nations Scientific Committee on the Effects of Atomic Radiation and the National Academy of Sciences Committee on the Biological Effects of Ionizing Radiations, are actively involved in evaluating these studies and estimating biological risk from radiation.

Of all late effects, the induction of cancer and genetic damage are the most important. The lifetime risk of a fatal cancer (any type) from a single uniform exposure to the total body depends on the age at the time of exposure and the dose and dose rate. NCRP report 116 (1993) takes into account both factors and estimates the fatal cancer risks (probabilities) from 1 Sv radiation exposures as given in Table 15.2.

Information on genetic damage has been deduced mostly from results obtained in experiments with Mediterranean fruit flies (*Drosophila*) and laboratory mice. The present estimate of the doubling dose for genetic effects (the dose needed to double the natural incidence of a genetic or somatic anomaly) is in the range of

Table 15.1.   Radiation Doses and Acute Effects

Stage	Dose Range (rad)	Symptoms
No acute effect	0–200 (0–2)[a]	Usually unobservable
1	150–400 (1.5–4)	Transient nausea and vomiting; some evidence of damage to hematopoietic system, recovering in 1–2 months
2	350–600 (5–6)	Severe damage to hematopoietic system; bone marrow transplant essential; survival chances moderate
3	550–1000 (5.5–10)	Gastrointestinal damage; severe nausea, vomiting, and diarrhea; very small chance of recovery; death follows in 10–24 days
4	1000 and above (10 and higher)	Confusion, shock, burning sensation; death follows within hours

[a]Values in parentheses are in Gy.

Table 15.2. Radiation Risk of Fatal Cancer to Various Populations

High Dose and High Dose Rate	Risk of Fatal Cancer
General population (all ages)	10×10^{-4} rem^{-1} or 10×10^{-2} Sv^{-1}
Working population (18 yr or older)	8×10^{-4} rem^{-1} or 8×10^{-2} Sv^{-1}
Low Dose and Low Dose Rate	
General population (all ages)	5×10^{-4} rem^{-1} or 5×10^{-2} Sv^{-1}
Working population	4×10^{-4} rem^{-1} or 4×10^{-2} (Sv^{-1})

60–160 rad (0.6–1.6 Gy). This may be an overestimate because recent data indicate that humans are less sensitive to genetic damage than the fruit fly. For radiation protection, NCRP Report 116 estimates a risk value for severe hereditary effects of 0.8×10^{-4} rem^{-1} (0.8×10^{-2} Sv^{-1}) for workers (18 years or older) and 1.3×10^{-4} rem^{-1} (1.3×10^{-2} Sv^{-1}) for the general population (all ages). As can be safely inferred from these data, carcinogenic effects of radiation are more significant than genetic effects. Total detriment from radiation for cancer induction and genetic damage is then determined by adding the two risks.

RADIATION EFFECTS IN THE FETUS

The embryo and fetus are more susceptible to radiation than the adult. Radiation during fetal life may not only cause fetal death and induce cancer, but also may produce various gross and behavioral abnormalities and malformations. The most sensitive stage for the production of these abnormalities is between 3 and 15 weeks after conception, and the most common abnormality in humans occurs in the central nervous system (mental retardation). Radiation studies of rodents during this interval suggest that doses as low as 5 rad (cGy) may produce gross congenital malformations. Below 5 rad, the main risk to a fetus is the increased probability of cancer, which at present is estimated to be two to three times that of an adult (i.e., 1×10^{-3} rem^{-1} or 1×10^{-1} Sv^{-1} for lifetime).

DIFFERENT RADIATION EXPOSURES AND THE CONCEPT OF EFFECTIVE DOSE OR EFFECTIVE DOSE EQUIVALENT

The general population is exposed to a variety of radiation sources, and the type and amount of exposed tissue also vary from source to source. How does one compare the risks from radiation under these circumstances? Recently (NCRP Report 116), a new concept called "effective dose" has been introduced for such purposes. I discuss the various sources of radiation exposure in the United States and then follow it with the definition of effective dose and related concepts.

Sources of Radiation Exposure

In the United States, people are exposed to radiation for a variety of reasons. The foremost source of radiation exposure in this regard and possibly with no benefit is the natural background radiation that is present everywhere and all the time. There is little that can be done to eliminate it. It arises from extraterrestrial and terrestrial sources. Cosmic rays and radionuclides produced by them (e.g., ^{14}C) are the primary source of extraterrestrial radiation. Its amount is lowest at sea level and it increases with altitude. Terrestrial sources of background radiation are long-lived radionuclides such as ^{226}Ra (and daughter radionuclides such as ^{222}Rn, as discussed in Chapter 2) and ^{40}K that are present in minute but varying quantities everywhere on earth. The radionuclide ^{40}K is incorporated in the food chain and as a result is also present in small amounts in humans. The second source of radiation exposure is technology based. Artificial sources that are used in medicine or industry (nuclear weapons and nuclear energy) and natural sources that produce exposure as a result of gainful or pleasure-enhancing activity (e.g., uranium mining and cigarette smoking) fall under this category.

Methodology for Comparison of Different Exposures

How does one compare radiation risks from a variety of radiation exposures? It is not a straightforward proposition because many factors, such as type of radiation, amount and type of tissue irradiated, age at the time of irradiation, sex, dose, and dose rate, are considered. Recently, the NCRP (Report 116) considered most of these factors when exposure of the general population or radiation of occupational workers is involved and developed the following methodology. This analysis is not applicable to radiation exposure of a patient where risk and benefit analysis has to be done on an individual basis.

First, estimate the average dose D (rad or Gy) to a tissue or tissues. Second, determine the equivalent dose, H_T, by multiplying the average dose D with the appropriate radiation weighting factor, w_R, as discussed earlier (equation [1]). Third, determine the effective dose by using tissue weighting factors as described below. In the case of internally deposited radionuclides, two other terms, committed equivalent dose and committed effective dose, are used. This is to account for a wide range of the half-lives (from seconds to thousands of years) of radionuclides that exists in nature. These are also defined below.

EFFECTIVE DOSE, EFFECTIVE DOSE EQUIVALENT, AND TISSUE WEIGHTING FACTORS

Because the risk estimates given in Table 15.2 are for a uniform total body irradiation, risks from a partial body or inhomogeneous irradiation have to be adjusted appropriately. For this purpose, tissue factor, w_T, which attempts to take into account the variations in radiosensitivity of different tissues (averaged over age and sex in a given population), are used. The currently recommended tissue factors by NCRP are given in Table 15.3. The NRC regulations still use the conventional weighting factors. These are also given in Table 15.3. By using NCRP tissue weighting factors, one determines an effective dose, E, for a given irradiation condition (exposure). However, by using the NRC tissue weighting factors, one determines the effective dose equivalent, or ede. The effective doses (or edes) are then used to compare the risks from exposures under different conditions such as exposure from background radiation versus radiation exposure from medical procedures to the U.S. population. An exposure with higher effective dose (or ede) proportionally carries a higher risk. The effective dose (or ede, in which case NRC

Table 15.3. Tissue Weighting Factors, W_T, for Different Tissues or Organs According to NCRP and NRC Regulations

	NCRP Report 116	NRC
Gonads	0.20	0.25
Red bone marrow	0.12	0.12
Colon	—	0.12
Lung	0.12	0.12
Stomach	—	0.12
Bladder	—	0.05
Breast	0.15	0.05
Liver	—	0.05
Esophagus	—	0.05
Thyroid	0.03	0.05
Skin	0.01	0.01
Bone surface	0.03	0.01
Remainder	0.30	0.05

tissue weighting factors are used) is defined as follows:

$$E = \sum w_T H_T \qquad [2]$$

where Σ is summation over all irradiated tissues and organs, T.

COMMITTED EQUIVALENT DOSE AND COMMITTED EFFECTIVE DOSE

Calculations of effective doses from internal sources of radiation due to ingestion or inhalation of radionuclides pose a problem, particularly those with half-lives longer than 100 years. Because radiation exposure beyond the average life span of a human (about 70 years) is meaningless, the dose calculation of Chapter 7 has to be modified for long-lived radionuclides (of course, none of these are used in nuclear medicine but are encountered as background). For such cases, the NRC defined two other terms, committed equivalent dose to a tissue and committed effective dose. The committed equivalent dose to a tissue from an internal source of a radionuclide, $H_T(\tau)$, is the integral of the dose rate (see Chapter 7, equation [2]) for time interval τ (instead of 0 to infinity). The committed effective dose from a radionuclide, $E(\tau)$, then is the tissue weighted sum of $H_T(\tau)$ to all tissues as given by equation (2). τ denotes a specified period of exposure on which integration of the dose rate has to be performed (τ will vary with age at the time of intake for an individual). For a member of the general public (all ages), it is taken as 70 years and for a radiation worker (18 years or older), 50 years. In the case of a particular individual such as a radiation worker, his or her age at the time of intake will determine τ.

The NCRP (Report 116) recommended limits on exposures to the general public and workers based on the effective dose that combines doses from both external and internal sources. These have been adopted by the NRC, again with a few modifications, and are given in the next chapter.

EFFECTIVE DOSES IN NUCLEAR MEDICINE AND COMPARISON WITH OTHER SOURCES OF EXPOSURE

In nuclear medicine, two types of populations are exposed to radiation, patients who receive radiopharmaceuticals for medical benefit and radiation workers such as technologists, physicists, and physicians. How does medical exposure of the U.S. population compare with other sources of exposure such as background? Table 15.4 gives the average annual effective doses from various sources of radiation to the U.S. population. Nuclear medicine procedures give less than 5% of the effective dose due to background radiation. Among all sources of medical exposure, its contribution is about 26%. From both points of view, nuclear medicine procedures, considering the health benefits they provide, are a minor factor in the total effective dose received by the U.S. population. What about radiation exposure to nuclear medicine personnel? It is estimated to be about 100 mrem (1 mSv) per year for diagnostic radiology and nuclear medicine personnel and is the lowest among radiation workers such as uranium mine workers (23 mSv), nuclear power personnel (5.5 mSv), radiation therapy workers (1.7 mSv), and special radiology procedures (18 mSv).

Effective dose is primarily used to compare ra-

Table 15.4. Estimated Average Annual Effective Doses From Various Sources of Radiation Exposure to the U.S. Population

Source	Effective Dose (yr in mSv)
Background (all types)	3.0 (300)[a]
Smoking (Po-210)	2.8 (280)
Medical procedures	
Total	0.54 (54)
Nuclear medicine only	0.14 (14)
Consumer products	0.07 (7)
Occupational	0.009 (0.9)
Others	<0.002 (0.2)

[a]Values in parentheses are in mrem.

diation risks to the general population or a group of radiation workers. However, as a guideline, these can also be used to compare risks to patients from different medical procedures. For example, to compare risks from two nuclear medicine procedures, one first calculates the radiation dose (rad or Gy) to various organs from the two procedures, as was done in Chapter 7. Radiation doses are then converted into equivalent doses (rem or Sv) by multiplying with radiation weighting factor (1.0 in this case). Radiation doses to various organs from the two procedures are then multiplied by their tissue weighting factors (Table 15.3) and added together to obtain the effective dose (or effective dose equivalent) for each procedure. The procedures with higher effective doses carry a proportionally higher risk. For example, the radiopharmaceuticals ^{67}Ga citrate and ^{99m}Tc-labeled phosphate compounds give effective doses of 22 mSv and 5 mSv, respectively, which means that gallium imaging carries about four times more risk than bone imaging. This is a different, but more realistic, conclusion than if we compared either the total body or critical organ doses listed in Table 7.5 for the two procedures. In the case of evaluation of risk to a particular individual, effective dose has to be modified by factors such as age and/or sex of the individual at the time of exposure.

Key Points

1. Biological effects of radiation are preceded by a variety of physiochemical processes.

2. Biological effects are dependent on total dose, dose rate, LET of radiation, type and amount of tissue irradiated, and presence or absence of chemical modifiers in the irradiated tissue.

3. Two kinds of biological effects, stochastic and nonstochastic, are observed. Nonstochastic effects are observed at high doses and high dose rates and have a threshold and the severity of the effect depends on the dose. Stochastic effects are assumed not to have a threshold and the probability of occurrence is related to the dose and not the severity of the effect. At low doses and dose rates (most diagnostic exposures), radiation risk to an exposed individual primarily comes from stochastic effects.

4. For the same dose, biological effect may be different for different radiations and different tissues. The two terms, equivalent dose and effective dose, are designed to account for these two variables of the biological effect.

5. In humans, induction of cancer and genetic damage are the two deleterious effects of radiation that are of major concern.

6. Medical radiation exposure to the U.S. population is only 5% of that received from background radiation. Exposure from nuclear medicine procedures is only 25% of all medical radiation exposure to the U.S. population.

Questions

1. List the various stages in the development of radiation injury.

2. For the same radiation dose, what are the other factors that can modify the biological effects or their intensity?

3. Generally, below what dose are acute effects not observable?

4. Name the most common late biological effect and give its probability of occurrence after 1 rem of total body irradiation at low dose rate to a general population.

5. What is the most sensitive period during pregnancy for the development of a fetal abnormality?

6. What factor relates absorbed dose to equivalent dose or dose equivalent?

7. What is tissue weighting factor and why is it needed?

8. Effective doses from an internally absorbed radionuclide have to be modified. Why? How?

16 Methods of Safe Handling of Radionuclides and Pertaining Rules and Regulations

Any use of radionuclides is fraught with the danger of inadvertently exposing an individual to radiation and therefore to its attendant hazards. This is especially true in the nuclear medicine laboratory where large amounts of unsealed radioactive sources are routinely handled. Each time a generator is milked, a radiopharmaceutical dose is drawn or injected, or a scan is performed on a patient, there is the possibility of exposure and contamination to the user (technician, physicist, or physician) and to the environment. Keeping this in mind, this chapter has two broad objectives: to describe the principles for minimizing radiation exposure and provide some practical ways in which an individual user can minimize exposure to oneself and fellow workers and reduce contamination of the environment and to give an overview of the extent and the scope of the pertinent rules and regulations that govern the use of radionuclides in nuclear medicine. For detailed descriptions, reading of the actual and most recent documents (the rules and regulations in this area are subject to periodic changes) is recommended.

PRINCIPLES OF REDUCING EXPOSURE FROM EXTERNAL SOURCES

Hazard from external radiation sources is measured in terms of exposure. Exposure is a measure of the ability of radiation to produce ionization in air. The unit of exposure is the roentgen (R), that level of radiation which produces ionization in air in the amount of 2.58×10^{-4} coulomb/kg of air. A milliroentgen (mR) is one thousandth of a roentgen. The SI units of exposure are simply coulomb/kg. Therefore, 1 coulomb/kg = 3876 R.

If the exposure is known at a given point, one can calculate the absorbed dose to a person at that point by multiplying the exposure by a term known as "f" factor. For muscle and soft tissue, f factor is close to unity. Therefore, for purposes in nuclear medicine, we may assume that exposure is more or less equivalent to the absorbed dose, which is equal to dose equivalent, that is, 1 R (1/3876 Coulomb/kg) $\equiv$ 1 rad (0.01 Gy) $\equiv$ 1 rem (0.01 Sv).

The principle of reducing exposure to radiation from sources outside the body (x- and γ-ray emitting radionuclides only) can be summed up in three equally important words: time, distance, and shielding.

Time

Because the total radiation dose, whether to the total body or part of the body, is directly proportional to the time of exposure, it is extremely important to spend as little time as possible near x- or γ-ray-emitting radionuclide sources. This requires forethought and precaution by the user. For example, when eluting a ^{99}Mo generator, one should not stand near it while the elution is in progress. When injecting a dose to a patient, one should locate the vein first and then take the syringe containing the radionuclide dose out of the leaded syringe carrier. However, rushing through a procedure is definitely not suggested here; if one has to repeat a procedure because of haste, total exposure time will be doubled.

Distance

Radiation dose to the body from a small external source varies inversely with the square of the distance of the source from the body (i.e., if we increase the distance from a source of radiation by a factor of 2, the radiation dose will drop by a factor of 4). Therefore, one should use a cart with a long handle when carrying very hot (> 50 mCi) radionuclide sources emitting high-energy γ-rays (> 300 keV) from one place to another, even though these sources are shielded. When radionuclide sources that are moderate in activity ($\approx$ 10 mCi) are hand-carried, the source should be held away from the body.

In drawing a dose for injection, use a syringe large enough so that it is no more than half-full when the desired volume is added and handle it from the unfilled area. If it is necessary to work with hot sources for long periods of time, then one should seriously consider the use of various remote-control tools available for picking up a radioactive vial or pipetting a radioactive solution.

Shielding

γ- and x-rays can be effectively shielded using thick containers, bricks, or partitions made of lead. Mirrors should be used for viewing behind lead partitions. The amount of actual shielding needed to reduce exposure to a minimal level depends on the amount of radioactivity to be shielded and the energy of the γ-rays. Use of a syringe lead shield to reduce exposure during radiopharmaceutical injection is essential in view of the ALARA ("as low as reasonably acceptable") principle. However, lead aprons worn in diagnostic radiology are not very effective in reducing exposure in nuclear medicine and therefore are not recommended.

The three variables, time, distance, and shielding, can be combined in a single formula that gives the exposure from a small radioactive source:

$$E = \frac{n\Gamma}{d^2} \cdot e^{-\mu(\text{linear})\cdot x} \cdot t \qquad [1]$$

Here E is the exposure (R), n is the number of millicuries in the source, d is the distance (cm) of the point (at which exposure is desired) from the source, t is the time of exposure (hr), μ(linear) is the linear attenuation coefficient of the shielding material (cm^{-1}), and x is the thickness of the shielding material (cm). Γ^* is the exposure rate constant of the radionuclide and its units are R $\cdot$ cm^2/mCi $\cdot$ hr. For ^{99m}Tc, its value is 0.60. For other radionuclides of interest to nuclear medicine, its values are given in Appendix A.

EXAMPLES:

(1) Calculate the exposure in 1 minute to the tips of the fingers from a syringe held by the tips of the fingers and containing 15 mCi of ^{99m}Tc radioactivity (assume the distance of the radioactivity from the tips of the fingers is 3 cm).
In this case,

n = 15 mCi, Γ = 0.60 R $\cdot$ cm^2/mCi $\cdot$ hr

t = 1 minute = $\frac{1}{60}$ hour

x = 0 (no shielding, neglect absorption in the source)

d = 3 cm

---

*For radiation protection work, γ- or x-rays with energies less than 20 keV are not included in the calculation of Γ.

Substituting these values in equation (1),

$$E = \frac{15 \times 0.6}{3^2} \cdot e^{-\mu(\text{linear}) \cdot 0} \cdot \frac{1}{60} R$$

$$= 0.017 \text{ R} = 17 \text{ mR}$$

(2) Calculate the same exposure as in example 1 except this time the syringe is shielded by 1-mm-thick lead (μ(linear) = 25 cm^{-1}]. In this case, x = 1 mm = 0.1 cm and μ(linear) = 25 cm^{-1}.
All other factors are the same.
Therefore, using equation (1), we get

$$E = \frac{15 \times 0.6}{3^2} \cdot e^{-25 \times 0.1} \cdot \frac{1}{60} R$$

$$= 0.017 \, e^{-2.5}$$

$$= 0.017 \times 0.08 = 0.00136 \text{ R}$$

$$= 1.36 \text{ mR}$$

(3) A patient has been injected with 15 mCi of ^{99m}Tc radioactivity. Calculate the exposure to a technician who, on average, takes 30 minutes to perform the scan and stays at about 1 m away from the patient during this time. (Assume the radioactivity is localized in a small volume in the patient and that there is no attenuation in the patient.)
In this case,

n = 15 mCi, Γ = 0.60 R $\cdot$ cm^2/mCi $\cdot$ hr

d = 1 m = 100 cm

t = 30 minutes = 0.5 hours

x = 0 and μ(linear) = 0

Using equation (1),

$$E = \frac{15 \times 0.6}{100^2} \cdot e^{-0} \cdot 0.5 R$$

$$= \frac{15 \times 0.6 \times 0.5}{10,000} = 0.00045 \text{ R}$$

$$= 0.45 \text{ mR}$$

If the attenuation in the patient is also taken into account, the exposure will be further reduced, probably by a factor of 4.

These illustrative examples show the extent of the possible exposure in nuclear medicine. The other and very important source of exposure is the radionuclide generator.

AVOIDING INTERNAL CONTAMINATION

Internal contamination by a radionuclide is possible by three routes: penetration through skin, ingestion, and inhalation. To avoid ingestion or penetration through the skin, the following steps should be taken.

1. Wear coveralls or a laboratory coat and disposable gloves each time you handle a radioactive material. Remember that the gloves, once you handle a radioactive material, become contaminated. Because they are the easiest source of spread of contamination in the laboratory, discard them immediately after handling radioactive material. When handling highly radioactive material, it is wise to wear two pairs of gloves.

2. Do not eat, drink, or smoke in the radionuclide laboratory or pipette radioactive solutions by mouth. Before eating, when you have been handling radioactive compounds, wash your hands thoroughly.

3. Keep the area neat in which radionuclides are handled. Use a tray with absorbent liners on the bench to limit the spread of radioactive material in case of an accident while working with unsealed radioactive sources.

4. Because the bed sheets, pillows, and stretchers used when scanning patients may be contaminated as a result of a patient's saliva, blood, or urine, beware of this route of personal contamination.

Contamination by inhalation does not pose a great problem in nuclear medicine except in a few cases where radioactive gases are used or large amounts of radioiodine are handled. To avoid the contamination of the room by radioactive gases, such items should be stored under a fume hood and, during use, proper care should be taken to prevent these gases from escaping into the room. In the case of large amounts of radioiodine, all work should be performed under a fume hood if possible. When opening a vial containing high amounts of radioiodine-labeled compounds, the vial should be extended away from you. In the administration of therapeutic doses of ^{131}I, allow patients to open the vial and drink the dose by themselves.

THE RADIOACTIVE PATIENT

A radioactive patient is an important source of radiation in nuclear medicine. Through penetrating radiations (x- or γ-rays), the patient can irradiate persons at a distance. Through physical contact or excretion and exhalation into the environment, the patient becomes a source of internal contamination. Presently, a patient has to be isolated in a private room if he or she has received more than 30 mCi (111 MBq) of radioactivity of a radionuclide or the measured dose equivalent at 1 m is less than 5 mrem/hr (0.5 Sv/hr). There are no such restrictions for radioactivity under this amount. However, because of ALARA, proper health physics principles, some of which have been described earlier, should be followed to keep the radiation exposure to a minimum level. Patients containing radioactivities of ^{131}I in amounts of 37–111 MBq (10-mCi) have a potential of exposing close relatives to more than 100 mrem (1 mSv) of effective equivalent dose (exposure limit for the general public). Therefore, appropriate instructions for limited contact with close family members and contamination containment should be provided to the patient.

A nursing mother is a special case of a radioactive patient that needs to be discussed separately. Because many radionuclides are excreted in milk, an infant dependent on his or her mother's milk may be exposed to undue risk. In such cases, all alternatives should be carefully weighed. For tests performed with technetium-labeled compounds, a simple rule of 2 days' cessation of breast feeding works well. For all of these compounds, the mother's radioactivity will decay by a factor of 1000 or more during this interval, and therefore little if any will be ingested by the infant. However, for tests using radionuclides such as ^{67}Ga, ^{111}In, ^{131}I, and ^{201}Tl, the situation is quite complex. Careful assessment and monitoring, coupled with several weeks of cessation, may be required to ensure that the infant is not exposed to undue risk.

RULES AND REGULATIONS
U.S. Regulatory Agencies

To ensure proper and safe use of radionuclides, a number of federal and state (called agreement states) agencies set standards for protection against radiation and issue regulations for production, transportation, possession, use, and disposal of radionuclides. The standards and regulations are primarily, but not entirely, based on the recommendation of the International Council on Radiation Protection and the National Council on Radiation Protection (NCRP). The U.S. Nuclear Regulatory Commission (NRC) is the federal agency most responsible for these regulations. These are published in the code of Federal Regulations under Title 10. The reader is urged to read this document, particularly parts 20 and 35, which are of direct relevance to nuclear medicine. NRC rules and regulations apply strictly only to the radionuclide produced by a nuclear reactor and not to radionuclides produced by a particle accelerator or cyclotron. The U.S. Food and Drug Administration is responsible for the regulations of the production of radiopharmaceuticals and their clinical or research use in humans. Two other federal agencies with shared responsibility with NRC are the Department of Transportation, which sets regulations for transport of radionuclides, and the Environmental Protection Agency, which sets regulations for the release of radionuclides in the atmosphere.

Exposure or Dose Limits: Annual Limit on Intake and Derived Air Concentration

Table 16.1 lists the exposure limits to various categories of persons. Both external and internal exposures are included, but exposure from natural sources is excluded from these limits. External doses are for tissues deeper than 1 cm (the deep dose equivalent) and the internal doses are committed effective doses. The dose limits are given as total effective dose equivalent and are based on the current NRC regulations. These are slightly different from those in NCRP Report 116. One major difference between the two is due to the use of different tissue weighting factors, as discussed in Chapter 15.

Normal annual exposures of workers in a clinical nuclear medicine department seldom exceed these limits and generally are about one-tenth of these limits.

Although these limits include internal exposure from radionuclides, calculations of committed effective dose and committed equivalent dose from different radionuclides are complicated (see Chapters 7 and 15). Therefore, to reduce the need of these calculations by individual user, two new entities that put limits on the intake of radionuclides based on the effective dose equivalent to a "reference man" (similar to the "standard man" of Chapter 7) are defined: the annual limit on intake (ALI) and the derived air concentration (DAC). These limits are published by the NRC for a large number of radionuclides and should not be exceeded.

ALI is defined as the amount of radioactivity of a radionuclide that if taken into the body would give a person (reference man) an effective dose equivalent of 50 mSv in 1 year. The ALI for ^{99m}Tc compounds is in millicuries and for ^{131}I in microcuries. These are relatively large limits and are never reached under normal and proper use of radiopharmaceuticals.

For airborne radioactivity, DAC is defined as ALI divided by the volume of air inhaled by a reference man in a working year (2.4×10^3 m³).

ALARA Principle

The limits in Table 16.1 are legal and are not to be exceeded at any time. However, these limits do not imply that radiation below this level is harmless or safe. The guiding principle in the radiation protection or health physics is that radiation doses should be "as low as reasonably achievable" (ALARA). This philosophy is mandated by law and therefore puts the onus on the user to reduce radiation levels in work places to as low a level as is economically and technologically feasible, even if these levels are well below the legal limits.

Types of Licenses

To practice nuclear medicine, a license issued by the NRC or an agreement state (New York City is one exception where a state has given its au-

Table 16.1.   Current NRC Maximum Permissible Annual Dose Limits

	Dose Limit (mSv)
Radiation (occupational) workers	
Total effective dose equivalent limits	50
Dose equivalent limits to tissues and organs	
Lens of eye	150
Skin, hands, and feet	500
Any other organ or tissue	500
General public	
Total effective dose equivalent	1
Embryo-fetus (entire pregnancy)	
Total effective dose equivalent	5

thority to a city) is required. The license can be for limited or broad use. A limited-use license is primarily designed for physicians in private practice or hospitals desiring to use radionuclides for specific purposes such as routine and well-established procedures. The broad-use license is issued to large medical centers and it allows, in addition to the use for routine procedures, a wider scope for research and development of new procedures. There are strict educational and training requirements to qualify for the license and a licensee takes upon him or herself to abide by all the conditions of a license.

Radiation Safety Committee and Radiation Safety Officer

One important requirement of the NRC is the establishment of a radiation safety committee (RSC) consisting of representatives from medical departments using radionuclides and administration. The RSC has the overall responsibility for the radiation safety under the license. It (or a licensee when an RSC is not mandated) designates a radiation safety officer (RSO), who is responsible for the actual implementation and monitoring of the safety program.

Personnel Monitoring

For the safety of nuclear medicine personnel, monitoring of radiation levels is required. This includes both external and internal monitoring.

EXTERNAL MONITORING

External monitoring is performed with small inexpensive dosimeters that can be worn on some part of the body externally. Three types of personnel monitors, film dosimeters, thermoluminescent dosimeters (TLDs), and pocket dosimeters, are used for external monitoring of radiation exposure.

Of these, the film dosimeter is the most common and economical, although not the most accurate. It consists of a small film enclosed in a plastic container with four windows covered with different radiation filters (e.g., no filter, aluminum, lead and aluminum, and cadmium and aluminum) to identify the nature and energy of the exposing radiation. The darkening on the film (film density; see Chapter 11) is related to the exposure level. It can measure radiation doses from 0.1 mGy to as high as 15 Gy. Film in

the dosimeter is normally changed each month. The old film is developed, exposure measured, and kept as a permanent record.

The TLD, as described in Chapter 8, is made of substances, such as LiF, that store in them the energy deposited by a radiation exposure for a long period of time and release it as light when they are subjected to heat. The amount of light produced is directly related to the radiation exposure. TLDs are accurate but expensive and, unlike a film dosi-meter, do not provide a permanent record.

Pocket dosimeters are small ionization chambers, Geiger-Mueller (GM) tubes, or semiconductor detectors that can measure and instantaneously display the radiation exposure. These are available for different ranges of exposures and used primarily for monitoring high-level exposures of short duration. These do not provide a permanent record.

INTERNAL MONITORING

Exposure from internal uptake of radionuclides as a result of occupational exposure is monitored through bioassays such as measurement of organ or total body uptake and urine or blood analysis for presence of radioactivity. Bioassay is required whenever ^{131}I is used for therapeutic purposes.

Receipt, Use, and Disposal of Radionuclides

A licensee is required to keep detailed records of the radioactivity received, the amount in storage, the amount used, and the amount disposed, if any, for all radionuclides he or she is authorized to possess. In no case should the total activity in possession exceed that allowed by the license.

Disposal of radionuclides for short-lived radionuclides such as ^{99m}Tc, ^{123}I, ^{67}Ga, ^{201}Tl, and ^{111}In is through decay in storage for a time period in which the radiation levels are reduced to less than two times the background. Excreta from radioactive patients can be released directly into the sewerage. Any other radioactive waste has severe restrictions on its release in sewerage or, in cases of gases such as ^{133}Xe, into the atmosphere. Of course, radioactive waste can always be transferred to an authorized recipient. Disposal of the old radionuclidic generators by returning it to the parent company is through such transfer.

Control and Labeling of Areas Where Radionuclides Are Stored and/or Used

The NRC mandates classification of areas as restricted and unrestricted. For restricted areas, it requires posting of warning signs, symbols, and labels denoting radiation. These include "Caution, Radiation Area" (> 5 mrem/hr or 0.05 mSv/hr dose equivalent at 30 cm from the source), "Caution, High-Radiation Area" (> 100 mrem/hr or 1 mSv/hr at 30 cm from the source), and "Caution, Radioactive Material" (in areas where radioactive material is stored or used and on containers of radioactive material).

Contamination Survey and Radiation-Level Monitoring

Depending on the level of radiation and the amount of radioactive material used, a licensee is required to monitor periodically the radiation levels and to wipe test for contamination of the areas where radiopharmaceuticals are handled or stored. A weekly survey of ambient radiation levels is performed with a calibrated GM counter. Calibration of the GM counter should be checked annually. Wipe tests are done by swabbing multiple areas with an absorbing material such as paper and counting them with a radiation detector (NaI(Tl) well-type counter if available). If contamination exceeds the regulatory limits, decontamination of the area is required. These limits are 0.01 μCi (370 Bq)/100 cm^2 for ^{99m}Tc and 0.001 μCi (37 Bq)/100 cm^2 for ^{131}I.

Receiving and Shipping (Transport) of Radioactive Packages

Monitoring of all packages labeled "radioactive material" is required. First, a visual inspec-tion to establish the integrity of the package is performed. Then, radiation levels at the surface and 1 m are measured, and a wipe test for possible surface contamination is performed. When the radiation levels exceed 200 mrem/hr (2 mSv/hr) at the surface or 10 mrem/hr (0.1 mSv/hr) at 1 m and/or the wipe test shows a reading of 22,000 decays per minute, prompt notification to appropriate authorities should be made.

To protect and warn of possible dangers to persons who may come in contact with a radioactive package, the Department of Transportation has issued specific rules and regulations for shipping radioactive packages. Three types of labels, depending on the surface level of radiation, are required: white-I, surface exposure less than 0.5 mR/h; yellow-II, surface exposure between 0.5 and 50 mR/hr and exposure at 1 m less than 1 mR/hr; and yellow-III, surface exposure between 50 and 200 mR/hr and exposure at 1 m between 1 and 10 mR/hr.

Accidental Radioactive Spills

Despite taking the necessary and appropriate precautions, accidents happen and a spill of radioactive material may occur. A radioactive spill is classified as minor (less than a milli-curie) or major (more than a millicurie). For major spills, the RSO has to be notified, who then investigates the incident and recommends corrective action.

In case of a spill, access to the area should be immediately restricted, the spill contained by using liquid absorbers or closing of the room in case of radioactive gases or vapors, and it should be followed by decontamination of the personnel involved and the area of spill.

Key Points

1. Radiation exposure in the nuclear medicine laboratory can result from both external and internal sources.

2. External exposure can be minimized by keeping ones distance from the radioactive source, spending minimum time necessary near a radioactive source, and shielding radioactive sources appropriately.

3. Internal contamination can be reduced by following proper laboratory procedures.

4. There are regulatory limits (Table 16.1) on exposure to radiation workers and the general public. There are no regulatory limits on radiation exposure to patients except that benefits outweigh the risk of a medical exposure.

5. Monitoring of the external exposure and internal uptake in certain circumstances of the nuclear medicine personnel is mandatory.

6. There are general rules and regulations for possessing, using, and disposing of radionuclides and some specific rules related to medical use of radionuclides. All persons working in nuclear medicine should be aware of these rules.

Questions

1. Which radionuclide with the following exposure rate constants (Γ) poses the most danger as an external source of radiation? (a) 2.0 R/mCi/hr, (b) 100 mR/mCi/hr, (c) 2.0 R/mCi/day, and (d) 1.0 R/mCi/min.

2. A patient who was treated with 100 mCi of radioiodine measured 10 mR/hr at 100 cm at the time of administration. By the next day, this measurement dropped to 2 mR/hr. How much radioactivity does the patient still have?

3. A radioactive syringe produces an exposure rate of 1 R/hr at a distance of 20 cm. Calculate the exposures of two persons who were working for 3 hours at 50 cm and 100 cm, respectively, from the syringe.

4. Which is the larger source of internal contamination, ingestion or inhalation?

5. What limits are currently imposed on the radiation exposure of a radiation worker, member of the general population, and a patient?

6. Does a film-type exposure dosimeter measure total effective dose equivalent?

Physical Characteristics of Some Radionuclides
of Interest in Nuclear Medicine

Table A.1. **Radiations Emitted in the Decay of ^{123}I ($\Gamma = 1 \cdot 53$ R $\cdot$ cm^2/mCi $\cdot$ hr); T$_{\frac{1}{2}}$ = 13 hr**

Number	Radiation (i)	Frequency of Emission (n$_i$)	Mean Energy (MeV) (E$_i$)
1	γ1	0.84	0.159
2	K conversion electron	0.13	0.127
3	L conversion electron	0.02	0.154
4	γ2	0.01	0.529
5	X-ray-K (α)	0.71	0.027
6	X-ray-K (β)	0.15	0.031
7	X-ray-L	0.13	0.003
8	LMM Auger electron	0.92	0.003
9	MXY Auger electron	2.19	0.001

Table A.2. **Radiations Emitted in the Decay of ^{131}I ($\Gamma = 2 \cdot 2$ R $\cdot$ cm^2/mCi $\cdot$ hr); T$_{\frac{1}{2}}$ = 8.1 days**

Number	Radiation (i)	Frequency of Emission (n$_i$)	Mean Energy (MeV) (E$_i$)
1	β1	0.02	0.069
2	β2	0.07	0.096
3	β3	0.90	0.192
4	γ1	0.03	0.080
5	K conversion electron	0.03	0.046
6	γ2	0.06	0.284
7	γ3	0.82	0.364
8	K conversion electron	0.02	0.330
9	γ4	0.07	0.637
10	γ5	0.02	0.723

From J Nucl Med 1975; (Suppl 10).

Table A.3.   Radiations Emitted in the Decay of ^{201}Tl (Γ = 0.47 R · cm^2/mCi · hr); T$_{\frac{1}{2}}$ = 73 hr

Number	Radiation (i)	Frequency of Emission (n$_i$)	Mean Energy (MeV) (E$_i$)
1	γ1	0.01	0.032
2	L conversion electron	0.21	0.018
3	M conversion electron	0.07	0.029
4	γ2	0.04	0.135
5	K conversion electron	0.10	0.052
6	L conversion electron	0.02	0.121
7	γ3	0.12	0.167
8	K conversion electron	0.18	0.084
9	L conversion electron	0.03	0.154
10	X-ray-K (α)	0.78	0.070
11	X-ray-K (β)	0.22	0.081
12	X-ray-L	0.46	0.010
13	KLL Auger electron	0.03	0.055
14	KLX Auger electron	0.02	0.066
15	LMM Auger electron	0.81	0.008
16	MXY Auger electron	2.44	0.003

Table A.4.   Radiations Emitted in the Decay of ^{133}Xe (Γ = 0 · 15 R · cm^2/mCi · hr); T$_{\frac{1}{2}}$ = 5.3 days

Number	Radiation (i)	Frequency of Emission (n$_i$)	Mean Energy (MeV) (E$_i$)
1	β1	0.02	0.075
2	β2	0.98	0.101
3	γ1	0.01	0.080
4	K conversion electron	0.01	0.044
5	γ2	0.36	0.081
6	K conversion electron	0.53	0.045
7	L conversion electron	0.08	0.076
8	M conversion electron	0.03	0.080
9	X-ray-K (α)	0.39	0.030
10	X-ray-K (β)	0.09	0.035
11	X-ray-L	0.08	0.004
12	Auger electrons	1.67	0.003

Table A.5.   Radiations Emitted in the Decay of ^{111}In ($\Gamma = 1 \cdot 9$ R $\cdot$ cm^2/mCi $\cdot$ hr); T$_{\frac{1}{2}}$ = 67.4 hr

Number	Radiation (i)	Frequency of Emission (n_i)	Mean Energy (MeV) (E_i)
1	Gamma 1	0.90	0.172
2	K conversion electron	0.09	0.145
3	L conversion electron	0.01	0.168
4	Gamma 2	0.94	0.247
5	K conversion electron	0.05	0.220
6	L conversion electron	0.007	0.243
7	K (α) X-ray	0.70	0.023
8	K (β) X-ray	0.14	0.026
9	L-X-ray	0.11	0.003
10	KLL Auger electron	0.11	0.019
11	KLX Auger electron	0.04	0.022
12	LMM Auger electron	0.99	0.002

Table A.6.   Radiations Emitted in the Decay of ^{67}Ga ($\Gamma = 0 \cdot 80$ R $\cdot$ cm^2/mCi $\cdot$ hr); T$_{\frac{1}{2}}$ = 78.1 hr

Number	Radiation (i)	Frequency of Emission (n_i)	Mean Energy (MeV) (E_i)
1	Gamma 1	0.033	0.091
2	Gamma 2	0.38	0.093
3	K conversion electron	0.28	0.084
4	L conversion electron	0.038	0.092
5	M conversion electron	0.013	0.093
6	Gamma 3	0.24	0.185
7	Gamma 4	0.025	0.209
8	Gamma 5	0.16	0.300
9	Gamma 6	0.04	0.394
10	K-X-ray	0.46	0.009
11	Auger electron	0.66	0.008

Quantity	CGS Units	MKS or SI Units	Conversion Factors[a] (CGS→ MKS)
Length	Centimeter (cm)	Meter (m)	0.01
Mass	Gram (g)	Kilogram (kg)	0.001
Time	Second (sec)	Second (sec)	1
Energy	erg	Joule (J)	10^{-7}
Radioactivity	Curie (Ci)	Becquerel (Bq)	3.7×10^{10}
Exposure	roentgen (R)	Coulomb/kilogram (C/kg)	2.58×10^{-4}
Absorbed dose	rad	Gray (Gy)	0.01
Dose equivalent	rem	Sievert (Sv)	0.01
Equivalent dose	rem	Sievert (Sv)	0.01
Effective dose	rem	Sievert (Sv)	0.01
Effective dose equivalent	rem	Sievert (Sv)	0.01

[a]To obtain results in the MKS system, multiply the CGS values by the conversion factor. To obtain results in the CGS system, divide the MKS values by the conversion factor.

Exponential Table

x	e^{-x}	x	e^{-x}	x	e^{-x}
0.00	1.00	0.22	0.80	0.60	0.55
0.01	0.99	0.24	0.79	0.65	0.52
0.02	0.98	0.26	0.77	0.693	0.50[a]
0.03	0.97	0.28	0.76	0.75	0.47
0.04	0.96	0.30	0.74	0.80	0.45
0.05	0.95	0.32	0.72	0.85	0.42
0.06	0.94	0.34	0.71	0.90	0.41
0.07	0.93	0.36	0.70	1.00	0.37
0.08	0.92	0.38	0.68	1.50	0.22
0.09	0.91	0.40	0.67	2.00	0.13
0.10	0.90	0.42	0.66	2.50	0.08
0.12	0.89	0.44	0.64	3.00	0.05
0.14	0.87	0.46	0.63	3.50	0.03
0.16	0.85	0.48	0.62	4.00	0.02
0.18	0.84	0.50	0.61	4.50	0.01
0.20	0.82	0.55	0.58	5.00	0.007

[a] See Chapter 3, p. 21.

Appendix D

Radionuclides of Interest in Nuclear Medicine

Radionuclide	Method of Production	Mode of Decay	Principal Photons (KeV)[a]	Half-life
Used clinically, mainly for diagnosis—generator				
^{99}Mo	Fission	β^-	740(14), 780(5)	67 hr
^{99m}Tc	Generator	IT	140(88)	6 hr
^{81}Rb	Cyclotron	EC, β^+	511(54)	4.6 hr
^{81m}Kr	Generator	IT	190(67)	13 sec
Used clinically, mainly for diagnosis—no generator				
^{51}Cr	Reactor	EC	320 (100)	27.8 days
^{67}Ga	Cyclotron	EC	93(40),184(24),296(22),388(7)	78 hr
^{111}In	Cyclotron	EC	173(89), 247(94)	67 hr
^{123}I	Cyclotron	EC	159(83)	13 hr
^{125}I	Reactor	EC	27–31(142)	60 days
^{133}Xe	Reactor	β^-	80(37)	5.3 days
^{201}Tl	Cyclotron	EC	69–80(94), 167(10)	73.1 hr
Used clinically, mainly for diagnosis—PET				
^{11}C	Cyclotron	β^+	511 (200)	20.4 min
^{13}N	Cyclotron	β^+	511 (200)	10 min
^{15}O	Cyclotron	β^+	511 (200)	2 min
^{18}F	Cyclotron	β^+, EC	511 (194)	110 min
^{68}Ga	Cyclotron	β^+, EC	511 (176)	68 min
Used clinically mainly for therapy				
^{32}P	Reactor	β^-	None	14.3 days
^{89}Sr	Reactor	β^-	None	52 days
^{131}I	Fission	β^-	364(82)	8.1 days
Used as standard source				
^{57}Co	Cyclotron	EC	122 (86)	270 days
^{137}Cs	Fission	β^-	660 (100)	30 yr

[a]Values in parentheses are % emission frequency. IT = isomeric transition; EC = electron capture.

Appendix E

Organ Masses of a Standard Man

Organ	Mass (g)
Total body	70,000
Bladder	509
Kidneys (both)	288
Liver	1833
Lungs	999
Ovaries	8.8
Pancreas	61
Skeleton with marrow	10,091
Spleen	176
Stomach	402
Testicles	38
Thyroid	20

Answers

Chapter 1

1. (a) 27.98; (b) 72.14 keV.

2. (a) 2.15, 7.11, and 59.40; (b) 1.19, 5.19, and 15.86 keV.

3. 1.24, 0.124, and 0.0124 angstrom.

4. 511 keV and γ-ray.

5. 2 (exact number is 2.52, one cannot create a fraction of an electron).

Chapter 2

1. Isotopes: $^3_2$He, $^4_2$He and $^{12}_6$C, $^{14}_6$C; isobars: $^3_1$H, $^3_2$He and $^{12}_6$C, $^{12}_7$N; isotones: $^3_1$H, $^4_2$He and $^{99}_{43}$Tc, $^{100}_{44}$Ru; and isomers: $^{99}_{43}$Tc, $^{99m}_{43}$Tc.

2. (a) Beta decay or isobaric transition; (b) positron emission or K capture; (c) electron emission; (d) alpha decay; and (e) gamma decay or isomeric transition.

3. 0.0062 and 0.57 MeV, respectively.

4. Excited state and not ionized (electron cancels the charge of one proton in the nucleus, and therefore the atom stays neutral.)

5. Yes, there are no laws against it, although it is very rare.

6. Extra amount of energy.

7. (a) 0.021 MeV; (b) 0.172 and 0.247 MeV; (c) β_2 (0.298 MeV with 0.014 frequency), β_3 (0.452 MeV with 0.797 frequency), and $\gamma_7 + \gamma_8$ (18.5% combined emission); and (d) x-rays of 70 (78%), 81 (22%), and 10 (46%) keV.

8. γ_1, 25% and 0%, and γ_2, 25% and 100% for radionuclide A and C, respectively; 100 keV for both.

9. A, 200 keV (1 hour half-life).

10. 100.

Chapter 3

1. (a) 2.7×10^{-4} mCi; (b) 0.01 MBq.

2. 370 MBq.

3. (a) 10^5; (b) 3.6×10^8.

4. (a) 131; (b) 92.5; and (c) 0.370 MBq.

5. (a) 146; (b) 134; and (c) 156.2 hours.

6. 3 hours.

7. 10,000.

8. 95.

9. ±180.

10. 20.

Chapter 4

1. Capture of neutrons in reactor-produced radionuclides causes an excess of neutrons in the nucleus. Conversion of a neutron into a proton through beta decay is the most convenient process for achieving stability in these nuclides. In accelerator-produced radionuclides, protons are in excess and conversion of a proton into a neutron through β^+ and/or electron capture is favored.

2. The amount of target material, the flux of neutrons or charged particles, the reaction cross section, and the half-life of the radionuclide to be produced.

3. For the same amount of desired radioactivity, carrier-free radionuclides have the least amount of that element or chemical present. Small amount is less toxic and gives high labeling-efficiency.

4. Parent of an almost ideal radionuclide, ^{99m}Tc, easy availability, inexpensive, little parent breakthrough, and rapid eluting method.

5. No, because of the presence of ^{99}Tc, which technically is a radionuclide but for all practical purposes is stable (half-life is 200,000 years).

6. Large parent breakthrough increases patient radiation dose without any additional benefit. It may also interfere in imaging.

7. 0.15 μCi (5.6 KBq) of ^{99}Mo for each mCi (37MBq) of ^{99m}Tc.

8. 4 GBq.

9. 0.125 GBq.

10. At 12.8-hour intervals (rule is four times daughter's half-life).

Chapter 5

1. Single γ emission with energy in 100- to 300-keV range, no particulate emission, short half-life.

2. (a) b; (b) a; and (c) c.

3. Method of administration, blood flow, protein binding, and extraction efficiency.

4. Hinders.

5. In such a case, the radionuclidic purity of the radionuclide will increase (improve) with time.

6. Pertechnetate and reduced technetium.

7. By reacting with a reducing agent, oxygen decreases the amount of reducing agent needed for pertechnetate reduction.

8. Common examples: ^{99m}Tc-sulfur colloid, ^{99m}Tc-phosphate compounds, ^{99m}Tc-sulfur colloid, ^{201}Tl-thallous chloride, blood proteins or red cells appropriately labeled, ^{99m}Tc-DMSA, ^{99m}Tc-MAA, ^{99m}Tc-HIDA, ^{123}Iodide, ^{99m}Tc-sulfur colloid, ^{67}Ga-citrate, ^{123}I-amphetamines.

9. The FDA approves the human use of radiopharmaceuticals, and the NRC regulates the use of these radiopharmaceuticals from a general radiation safety perspective.

10. 15 days.

Chapter 6

1. 1-MeV α particle, 1-MeV electron, 50-keV x-ray, 400-keV γ-ray, and 1-MeV x-ray.

2. Mass, energy, and charge of the particle and the density of the interacting medium.

3. (a) Density of the medium; (b) no.

4. 5.8, 0.87, and 0.15 cm, respectively.

5. When gamma energy is close to the binding energy of electrons in the inner shells of the interacting atoms.

6. 71, 167, and 200 keV, respectively.

7. μ(linear) of water $= \mu$(linear) of ice/density of ice $= \mu$(linear) of steam/density of steam.

8. 67% transmitted and 33% interactions.

9. Of the 33% interactions, 26.4% photoelectric and 6.6% Compton.

10. 1.02 MeV.

Chapter 7

1. 3.5 Gy, 1.2 mGy, and 50 mGy, respectively.

2. Radiations emitted and their energies, dosage of radioactivity administered, absorbed fraction in the case of γ-rays, and the effective half-life.

3. Biological data.

4. Same.

5. Different because the absorbed fraction will be different in the three cases.

6. Energy of γ-ray, size and shape of the target organ, and distance between the source and the target organ.

7. $\tilde{A} = 1.44 x f x A_0 \times T_{\frac{1}{2}}(\text{eff})$.

8. S factor contains in it all the required physical data of a radionuclide. To calculate the radiation dose, one only needs the biodistribution data (cumulative radioactivity). S factors are calculated for a standard man; therefore, these cannot be used for a specific patient who may be quite different from a standard man, as in the case of children.

9. (a) Yes; (b) brain, being the farthest, will receive the least amount of radiation dose.

10. Gallium citrate.

Chapter 8

1. Linear attenuation coefficient and thickness of the sensitive material of the detector. It allows reduction of either radiation dose or imaging time.

2. Inversely. The shorter the dead time, the higher the count rate for which a detector can be used.

3. Proportional counters; however, these are not used in nuclear medicine.

4. Because the current produced by the interaction of a single radiation is too small to be detected by an ionization chamber.

5. About 60,000 counts per minute.

6. (1) GM counter; (2) NaI(Tl) scintillator detector; (3) dose calibrator; and (4) Ge(Li) detector.

7. High linear attenuation coefficient for γ-ray energies used in nuclear medicine, high light output, short dead time, inexpensive, and easy availability in large sizes.

8. To select pulses in a given range.

9. Narrowing the window will decrease the observed count rate.

10. 13, 14, and 16%, respectively. The detector with 13% energy resolution is the best.

Chapter 9

1. Either by using a large-area detector or by decreasing the distance between the source and the detector. No, it does not depend on the type of the detector. This gives the maximum geometric efficiency.

2. Decay rate and the observed count rate differ because of the overall detection efficiency. Decay rate of a sample is generally higher than the observed count rate.

3. Yes, unless this is taken into account by some other means.

4. Because of short range of beta particles.

5. 4π.

Chapter 10

1. Unknown shape and size of radionuclidic distribution in the body makes it difficult to correct for the attenuation and scattering of γ-rays.

2. By allowing the rejection of scattered γ-rays.

3. To select a well-defined field of view. Lead is a high atomic number and high-density material and is inexpensive. Other high atomic number and high-density materials (e.g., gold) are comparatively expensive.

4. Compromise between efficiency and the uniformity of response in the thyroid gland.

5. These had no capability for fast dynamic studies.

Chapter 11

1. Intrinsic spatial resolution and intrinsic efficiency.

2. More light will improve the energy resolution of the scintillation camera. This will improve the intrinsic spatial resolution and the rejection of more scattered γ-rays.

3. (a) Parallel hole; (b) converging; (c) diverging; and (d) pinhole.

4. The intensity should be decreased.

5. More bits will be needed and higher speed will be desirable.

Chapter 12

1. An improvement by a factor of 2 in resolution will decrease the sensitivity by a factor of 4. Therefore, sensitivity of the new collimator will be 12,500 cpm.

2. FWHM is best suited to study the relationships with various parameters of an imaging device. Point-spread function or modulation transfer function give most general and complete descriptions of the spatial resolution of an imaging device. Good for comparison of diverse imaging devices. Resolution phantoms, such as parallel bars, are good to monitor gross changes in spatial resolution of an imaging device and therefore used in quality control.

3. 14.14, 11.18, and 10.05 mm, respectively.

4. Because of edge packing, localization of interaction of a γ-ray in this area of the crystal is not very accurate.

5. Mislocalization.

6. (A) Yearly; (b) daily; (c) weekly; (d) yearly; and (e) daily.

Chapter 13

1. 10%.

2. Radiopharmaceuticals for tumor detection have higher contrast than those used for blood flow in the brain. Higher contrast means higher detectability.

3. Large-area and multiple-head scintillation camera have higher sensitivity that can be used to increase the detectability or to reduce the study time.

4. The contrast in nuclear medicine is much higher than that in computed tomography, but the spatial resolution in computed tomography is much better than that in nuclear medicine.

Chapter 14

1. In general, a 360° angle improves the result in SPECT, but when an organ is located near the surface (e.g., heart), a 180° angle is preferable. No.

2. Increase in the sensitivity. More rigorous quality control.

3. Because small errors in scintillation camera response are magnified during the reconstruction process.

4. Field (volume) of view in SPECT is not cylindrical and attenuation cannot be easily corrected.

5. The shorter the resolving time, the lesser the accidental counts in the detector pair.

Chapter 15

1. Energy deposition, energy transfer to other molecules, chemical reactions, and production and expression of the damage.

2. Dose rate, type of radiation, type and amount of irradiated tissue, presence of chemical modifiers, and biological variation.

3. Under 200 rads (2 Gy).

4. Cancer, 0.0005 excess mortality.

5. Between 3 and 15 weeks after conception.

6. Radiation weighting factor (quality factor).

7. Biological risk from the same dose to total body and individual organs is different. Tissue weighting factors make risk comparison for different type of exposure (total body versus an organ) possible.

8. The normal life span of humans is about 70 years, but many radionuclides have half-lives in thousands of years.

Chapter 16

1. d.

2. 20 mCi.

3. 0.48 and 0.12 R, respectively.

4. Ingestion.

5. 5 rem (50 mSv) and 0.1 rem (1 mSv).

6. No, it basically measures dose at a specific point.

Suggestions for Further Reading

1. Johns HE, Cunningham JR. The physics of radiology. 4th ed. Springfield, IL: Charles C Thomas, 1983.
2. Sorenson JA, Phelps ME. Physics in nuclear medicine. 2nd ed. New York: Grune & Stratton, 1987.
3. Sandler MP, Coleman RE, Patton JA, et al. Diagnostic nuclear medicine. 3rd ed. Baltimore: Williams & Wilkins, 1996;I.
4. Loevinger R, Budinger TF, Watson EE. MIRD primer for absorbed dose calculations. rev ed. New York: Society of Nuclear Medicine, 1997.
5. Craft BY. Single-photon emission computed tomography. Chicago: Year Book Medical Publishers, 1986.
6. Beir V. Health effects of exposure to low levels of ionizing radiation. Washington, DC: National Research Council, National Academy Press, 1990.
7. Shapiro J. Radiation protection—a guide for scientists and physicians. 2nd ed. Cambridge, MA: Harvard University Press, 1988.

Index

Page numbers in *italics* denote figures; those followed by a t denote tables.